ORTHOPEDICS AND SPINE

Strategies for Superior Service Line Performance

MARSHALL K. STEELE, MD

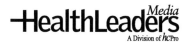

Orthopedics and Spine: Strategies for Superior Service Line Performance is published by HCPro, Inc.

Copyright © 2009 HCPro, Inc.

All rights reserved. Printed in the United States of America.   5   4   3   2

ISBN: 978-1-60146-631-0

HCPro, Inc., provides information resources for the healthcare industry. HCPro, Inc., is not affiliated in any way with The Joint Commission, which owns the JCAHO and Joint Commission trademarks.

Marshall K. Steele, MD, Author

Debra Beaulieu, Editor

Rick Johnson, Executive Editor

Matt Cann, Group Publisher

Doug Ponte, Cover Designer

Mike Mirabello, Graphic Artist

Genevieve d'Entremont, Copyeditor

Karen Holmes, Proofreader

Matt Sharpe, Production Supervisor

Susan Darbyshire, Art Director

Jean St. Pierre, Director of Operations

Advice given is general. Readers should consult professional counsel for specific legal, ethical, or clinical questions. Arrangements can be made for quantity discounts. For more information, contact:

HCPro, Inc.

75 Sylvan Street, Suite A-101

Danvers, MA 01923

Telephone: 800/650-6787 or 781/639-1872

Fax: 781/639-2982

E-mail: *customerservice@hcpro.com*

Visit HCPro at its World Wide Web sites: *www.hcpro.com* and *www.hcmarketplace.com*

Contents

Contents

                                            Orthopedics and Spine

   Orthopedics and Spine

About the Author

Marshall K. Steele, MD

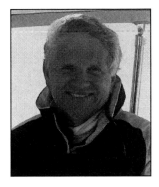

Marshall K. Steele, MD, has been involved in healthcare for more than 40 years in a variety of roles. He is a board-certified orthopedic surgeon and a member of the American Academy of Orthopedic Surgeons and the American Association of Hip and Knee Surgeons.

After finishing his orthopedic residency and serving in the Navy, he joined his father in orthopedic practice in Annapolis, MD, in 1977. By the time he retired from surgery in 2006, Steele had grown the practice into a 17-physician subspecialty orthopedic group that included programs in joints, spine, physiatry, sports medicine, foot/ankle, and hand.

Between 1996 and 2005, Dr. Steele also served in administrative roles at Anne Arundel Health Systems. As medical director of the operating room and surgical business development, he defined the core elements of excellence and created the model for patient-centric care, which he used to assist in the development of the organization's service lines—known as destination centers of superior performance—in joint, spine, and vascular surgery. These centers have proved to provide a superior patient and family experience, greater surgeon efficiency, higher market share, enhanced profitability, and national recognition.

In 2005, Dr. Steele founded Marshall Steele & Associates *(www.marshallsteele.com)*, which provides assessments, planning, implementation, and management of destination centers. The firm facilitates hospitals' long-term success by employing systems for electronic collection of patient-reported outcomes as well as benchmarking and trending of clinical, operational, financial, patient experience, and functional data.

Dr. Steele has written many articles on leadership and service-line development as well as one other book, *Sideline Help: A Guide for Immediate Evaluation and Care of Sports Injuries,* published by Human Kinetics in 1996. He can be reached at *marshallsteele@marshallsteele.com.*

Acknowledgments

This book was made possible because of significant contributions from several experts in orthopedic service-line implementation and success. My colleagues at Marshall Steele & Associates helped write various sections in their areas of expertise:

- Judy Jones, MS—vendor relationships, excellence

- Matt Reigle, MBA—implementation

- Craig Westling MS, MPH—operating room

- David Steele, MD, MBA—outcomes and management

- Lori Brady, RN—inpatient hospital care

- Ron Gaunt, RN—standardization, education

- Mary Ann Sweeney, PT—sports medicine

- Andrea Mastry, BA—marketing

- Patrick Vega, MS—spine programs, navigation

- Chad McClennan, MBA—patient experience

Others who made major writing contributions include:

- Thomas Graham, MD, director of the National Hand Center—hand centers

- Anthony Cirillo, FACHE, ABC—marketing

- Bill Munley, MBA—geriatric fracture care

Thanks to Debra Beaulieu, my editor, who put up with my constant changes and helped immeasurably in making this book better. Special thanks to my wife, Susan Steele, who has encouraged me to continue in this crusade of helping others make the changes that will transform healthcare.

Prologue

Since I finished medical school in 1971, much has changed and much has stayed the same. The technology has quickly outpaced my initial education, but even after nearly four decades, our culture of independence and reliance on individual performance persists. This has served us well in the past. However, the future will require a culture not of independence, but interdependence; not of individual performance, but of systems performance.

When I began orthopedic practice in Annapolis, MD, in 1977, most orthopedic surgeons were generalists. Half my practice came from the emergency room. The term "sports medicine" was just being introduced. Most of us thought of it as marketing and not substance. My father, Marshall Steele Jr., an orthopedic surgeon at the Naval Academy, spent most of his time caring for sports injuries. There were few civilian programs or centers in the country that could provide rapid access, accelerated rehabilitation, community education, and service for either young or old athletes.

In 1979, after a spending a few days in New York City with Dr. James Nicholas, one of the first sports doctors in the country, I returned anxious to create a sports medicine center in Annapolis. This resulted in the hiring of a fellowship-trained sports medicine orthopedist, sports-oriented physical therapists, and athletic trainers and physicians to provide education and support for our community athletic programs. Our success was enhanced by engaging many nonorthopedic physicians in both the care of athletes and coverage for local sports events.

Having the right people was vital, but creating systems (structure and processes) was equally essential. This included the development of a leadership team, a sports hotline number, a walk-in clinic, disease-specific educational tools, weekly articles for our local sports pages, and a guide for coaches in caring for injuries (*Sideline Help*). The incredible success of this center spawned my interest in service lines. Using this as a model, we developed additional programs for our practice in arthritis, spine, foot and ankle, and hand.

Despite the success of these programs, much was missing. We did not have coordinated care throughout the entire continuum, patient-reported outcomes were not being measured, operating room (OR) efficiency was lacking, and there was no organized system of care for joint and spine patients who were hospitalized after surgery. The end result was a mediocre hospital patient experience, fragmented care, more time in the lounge than the OR for surgeons, little hospital profitability, and outmigration of patients. A change was needed.

In the mid-1990s, I assumed several official administrative roles at Anne Arundel Medical Center in Annapolis. This included medical director of the OR and director of the surgical initiative (business development). As I contemplated what to do, two individuals were influential in my thinking: Dr. John Barrett, an orthopedic surgeon in Florida, and Regina Herzlinger, PhD, a Harvard professor and author of the landmark book *Market-Driven Health Care*. Their thoughts, combined with the support of hospital administrators Bill Bradel, Chip Doordan, and Sue Patton; Dr. Stephen Faust, an orthopedic colleague; and Dr. John Martin, a vascular surgeon, enabled us to transform the care we provided in joints, spine, and vascular surgery.

Specialized units, effective leadership structures, accountability, and creative delivery systems were created within the hospital. Our results were extraordinary: We improved the patient experience, family participation, quality of care, and profitability. The outmigration of the past became inmigration as we doubled market share and increased volumes up to sevenfold. Perhaps more importantly, these programs led to much better physician-physician and physician-hospital collaboration.

These successes were noted both domestically and internationally. Hundreds of hospitals visited us. However, post-visit surveys revealed that very few hospitals were able to implement this model themselves. A combination of being too busy, having little expertise in project management, no physician champion, and trying to improve incrementally seemed common roadblocks. These hospitals failed to realize that we were advocating transformation, not reformation of their old systems. Many of you reading this book run the risk of making the same mistake. When building a destination center, principles and people must be synchronized with structure and processes to achieve optimal results. I believe that this is how we can transform care.

I am so passionate about this that in 2005, I retired from surgery after 31 years and launched Marshall Steele & Associates as an implementation company to help hospitals and physicians make this transformation. Traveling the country has only strengthened my respect for and belief in the absolute desire of physicians, nurses, allied health professionals, and administrators to do the right thing. However, in assessing hospitals, I have learned that most still have the very traditional care and leadership model that was present in the 1970s when I started practice. Care is not patient- and family-centric by our new definition. The knowledge that patients and families possess to improve systems is not being used to make changes. It is rare that one person has or is responsible to manage all the metrics and care. Rather, management and care is done in silos by various departments and individuals. Even today, less than 5% of hospitals and physicians collect and aggregate information on whether their interventions actually helped their patients.

In an environment in which quality must be demonstrated and cost must be wrung out simultaneously, this will need to change. We have made a small dent. By spring 2009, our company had successfully implemented a program or two in more than 65 hospitals from coast to coast. These hospitals, ranging in size from 25 to 800 beds, are seeing the same great results that we experienced in Annapolis. However, there are 6,000 hospitals that need up to 20 or more programs apiece. It's a big task.

Healthcare is complicated, maybe the most complicated of any industry. There are many challenges in trying to transform care. Skeptics are everywhere, given the history of failed initiatives and broken promises. Changing the culture and the thinking of the individuals involved is just as vital for success as changing the care model.

Many well-intentioned individuals believe that physicians won't change. I disagree. However, you must create with them a compelling vision that they believe in and provide the data to support it.

This book does not contain all the answers. Rather, it is a combination of principles and experience of both the dedicated professionals in our company who are responsible for implementation of these programs as well as other colleagues with particular expertise in this area. These individuals are all acknowledged on p. ix.

One thing I have found is that there is a community of likeminded folks who are determined to make healthcare better. They are not waiting for the government to accomplish this. They understand that it can only be done by those of us on the front line. I welcome you to this community and to this journey. In the 1960s, my great-uncle Frank Laubach wrote a book, *Each One Teach One*. Using its principles, he taught much of the African continent how to read. He understood that nobody is smarter than everybody. As you read these pages, I hope they will spark new ideas. Please e-mail them to me at *marshallsteele@marshallsteele.com*. In so doing, you will become part of our community. I will share your ideas with others as I'll share theirs with you. I look forward to hearing from you.

Sincerely,
Marshall K. Steele III, MD

1

Overview of Orthopedics Today

Playwright George Bernard Shaw said, "The reasonable man adapts himself to the world. The unreasonable man tries to adapt the world. All progress is made by unreasonable men." I am hoping that those of you reading this book have some unreasonableness within you. This book is not about maintaining the status quo in medicine but changing it so that progress can be achieved.

Healthcare prices continue to rise and quality remains inconsistent. Nonetheless, we spend significantly more on healthcare than any other nation, and the U.S. healthcare system continues to receive poor grades on outcomes, quality of care, and efficiency.[1] Say what you might about how the grading is done, the trends are troubling. As Harvard economist Regina Herzlinger, PhD, pointed out in her 1997 book *Market-Driven Health Care: Who Wins, Who Loses in the Transformation of America's Largest Service Industry,* patients can find out more about the car they are going to buy than the results of the surgeon who has recommended surgery. Similar concerns were echoed by former speaker Newt Gingrich in his 2006 book *The Art of Transformation*: "Anything that is not personalized and responsive to changes in the individual, and which does not provide the customer with information about cost and quality, will rapidly find itself replaced by something that meets that standard of expectation."

Few organizations are able to meet this standard today. Tomorrow's patient will have even higher expectations of care and service. The public, the government, and the employers who pay for health insurance are getting restless. Transparency in cost and quality is emerging. Almost everyone agrees that healthcare and insurance are too expensive and that the system is fragmented and difficult to navigate. It is clear that the patient experience needs to be improved, quality needs to be more consistent, and errors must be reduced.

I like Yogi Berra's philosophy: "It's tough to make predictions, especially about the future." These days, we hear a lot of predictions, particularly when it comes to healthcare reform. President Obama has called the transformation of healthcare a moral and fiscal imperative. The hallmarks of his healthcare reform will be increased coverage and better services. He has stated that he wants to see payments for results, not just procedures; adoption of electronic medical records; and reduced reliance on expensive emergency department (ED) care. He wants healthcare to be more affordable by providing a public option for health insurance. This could signal the beginning of the end of employer-paid health insurance, which has already begun a steady decline. He expects to pay for all of this with increased efficiencies. Whether these changes become reality remains to be seen.

 Orthopedics and Spine

Is Healthcare a Commodity?

As a result of medical information being available to the public, some say medical care is becoming a commodity. The traditional doctor-patient relationship is all but extinct. Drugstores and other industries are providing medical care while you shop. Healthcare is no longer local. With the prevalence of information, the ease of travel, and hospitals wanting to care for patients coming from long distances, medical tourism has emerged. Medical tourism is not restricted to patients who travel from one country to another to receive medical care. More frequently, it is when patients travel from one county or one state to another. This has changed the hospital-community relationship. Community hospitals must step up or lose their elective base.

The number of patients needing healthcare, especially orthopedic services, is growing quickly; however, the number of orthopedic surgeons to care for them is not keeping pace. Orthopedic coverage in EDs is at risk in many hospitals. Each day, more and more hospitals are paying doctors to be on call. With margins below the 2.5% level for many hospitals, this becomes an additional burden.

Despite a wealth of uncertainty, several things are for sure. Hospitals and surgeons will be asked to do more with less. Costs must be reduced while quality improves. Transparency will become mandatory. There will be winners and losers. Those who accept the status quo and cling to the broken system of the past will not be the winners. The community hospital and its physicians must create a product and brand equal to or better than that of its larger competitors. It won't be enough for them just to think or say they are excellent; they will be asked to demonstrate their results. All the government can do is provide us with the right incentives. It cannot transform healthcare. That can be done only by those of us in the trenches.

Outlook for Surgeons

Surgeons will at least be able to count on having plenty of patients. For joint surgeons, the loss of reimbursement has been significant. In 1978, a total joint replacement reimbursement was $5,000. In 1994, it was reduced to $2,100, and by 2007 to $1,280. Whether surgeons will be fairly compensated and can increase their efficiency to handle more patients is unclear.

Given the economic pressures the country is facing, surgeon reimbursement is likely to decrease in real dollars rather than rise. Affected by this decline in reimbursement, surgeons will continue to find other avenues of income, such as surgical hospitals, ambulatory surgery centers, MRI, physical therapy, orthotics, and prosthetics. Providing these profitable services once provided by the hospital has created more stress on the hospital margins. Hospitals have asked the government to curb this activity. Just when we need closer physician-hospital relations to solve our issues, we have increased tension. Politicians have been debating the relative merits and pitfalls of having surgeons involved in this sector of healthcare. In this current environment, expect that debate to intensify. It is likely that more restrictions will be forthcoming.

Patients will continue to expect perfection from surgery. They feel that if we could put a man on the moon, we should certainly be able to provide nearly perfect healthcare. Physicians are held to a very high standard to do just that, and if they do not, they often find themselves in court. It is also unlikely that Congress will enact any significant tort reform, meaning that very costly defensive medicine and high malpractice premiums will continue.

With all this turmoil, many excellent orthopedic surgeons and large groups are now opting to become employed by hospitals. Compensation is usually based on relative value units worked. Employed surgeons still have significant governance in day-to-day practice decisions. I have observed this working quite well in many places. Goals can be more easily aligned. The orthopedic practice that I founded in 1977 has chosen this route. With the expected shortage of surgeons and national policy changes, this may be the best option for both parties. Whether employment becomes a success story for all involved will not be known for several years.

The Traditional Model

One of the major flaws with traditional medicine is that we don't have a com-prehensive system of coordinated patient-centric care. We have an "it depends" medicine. With specialization (a good thing) has come fragmentation. Everyone operates within silos. Primary care doctors have their systems and set of beliefs, as do surgeons, anesthesiologists, professional staff members, and so on. From their viewpoint, the care they are giving is excellent. However, this individualism, which to date is sacrosanct in healthcare, leads to multiple plans of care for the same condition.

Consider that for a procedure as straightforward as a total joint replacement, there could be as many as 10 care plans for a patient in the same hospital, depending on which professionals are involved. Having that many choices is not a good idea, even if they are evidence based. Operating within these silos can be costly and potentially harmful to the patient. It reduces efficiency for the staff while increasing the risk of error.

Henry Ford did not reduce the costs and improve the quality of his cars by improving individual performance. He did it by developing a system that was focused and repeatable. This did not result in incremental improvement but a transformation. Changing the fragmented, individualized practice we have used in this country for the past 100 years will not be easy. Our profession is dominated by professionals who often resist any thought of standardization as an encroachment on their independence. But incremental improvements won't get us to where we need to be. We need a transformation.

Tomorrow, with transparency and access to knowledge, patients, employers, payers, and physicians will be able to find out who has succeeded in making this transformation. They will seek out those institutions and physicians that can demonstrate superior performance. Patients will drive past one hospital after another to seek care at these institutions. Physicians and nurses will seek them out as the best places to work. They will become branded as destination centers. It can be done. It is being done. You can do it.

                                    Orthopedics and Spine

Destination Centers of Superior Performance

Surgeons are beginning to realize that their reputations are tied to the hospital-patient/family experience. Therefore, it is vital that they improve the care and experience of patients. Hospitals and surgeons must create a common vision for great patient care. One solution that has proven itself very effective is to create sophisticated service lines, which we like to call destination centers of superior performance. We take the best of traditional care and management—highly trained and qualified people—combine it with the needs of our patients—great experience and outcomes—and build it into a system of care. This is done by having the physicians and hospitals come together to create systems that are patient-centric and cost-effective.

The service line approach to orthopedic care represents a huge opportunity to resolve these challenges and more. "Service line" is a term borrowed from manufacturing industries that promote product lines. Similarly, hospital service lines seek to organize care delivery by disease processes, assemble dedicated clinicians and staff members to handle the entire care process, and coordinate with overlapping service lines.

I recently had the opportunity to explain this business approach to a teacher friend of mine: One service line, such as oncology, equates to language arts; another service line, such as cardiovascular, equates to mathematics; women's services equates to biology; and so on. Without service lines, one teacher would need to teach every subject. Can it be done? Sure. But would a great English teacher be as good at teaching science as a great science teacher? Maybe not.

This concept in healthcare was brought to my attention in the 1990s through the work of Regina Herzlinger, mentioned previously, who studied healthcare and determined that hospitals and patients would be much better off if hospitals and doctors developed efficient niche service lines, which she called "focused factories." Although the term "factory" offended many healthcare workers, who conjured up images of patients traveling down an assembly line, Herzlinger brought to light the notion that patients are better served in a specialty environment.

Many clinicians find that they are more effective in a service-line environment. For example, nurses working in the traditional model of care may find it difficult to provide patients the personal attention they need, as they are saddled with complexity, inconsistencies, inefficiencies, and paperwork. Some have told me they feel as though they are professionals on a team, not part of a professional team. A professional, specialized team, in contrast, is able to deliver care that is more efficient for physicians and clinical staff members and more personalized for patients.

Herzlinger's book and other articles at that time spurred interest in developing service lines across the country. Unfortunately, most hospitals focused on advertising service lines, not creating patient-centric care or implementing the core elements of excellence that we advocate in this book. They failed to create the structure and processes that would create a unique experience for patients, an effective work environment for physicians and staff members, as well as a system to manage for ongoing improvement. Without a great product, the dollars spent on advertising were wasted. Some even thought the service-line approach didn't work. Approaching the service line purely from the advertising side does not work. You need to create a unique product and measure your results. Then you can tell the public what differentiates you and why patients should seek care from your physicians and institution.

Opportunities abound

Because of the many systems and specialties linked to orthopedics, there are several potential types of orthopedic service lines in the inpatient and outpatient arenas. Depending on your organization's areas of expertise, you could offer one, two, or a full array of orthopedic service lines. As my principle expertise is in the creation of total joint replacement and spine centers, I will use this model as a frequent point of reference throughout the book. Although the concepts I provide generally apply to all orthopedic subspecialties, we will discuss the nuances of components including joint surgery, spine surgery, fracture care, arthritis care, sports medicine, and more in Chapter 10.

Service line development in musculoskeletal care is the perfect place to start. Primary hip replacements are expected to increase in demand by 174% by 2030, and primary knee replacements by 673%. Hip revisions are expected to increase by 137%, and knee revisions by 600%. Nationally, back and neck pain represent the second most frequent reason patients see a doctor (the first is the common cold). More than 13 million people annually visit physician offices for back pain. Chronic back pain accounts for 15% of all sick leaves and is the leading cause of adult disability.

New surgical technologies for the spine have enabled this market to experience over 10% growth per year during the past decade. Geriatric fractures are on the rise, and many can be prevented. Sports medicine, a term used only as a marketing tool when I started practice, is now the preferred path for young orthopedists and patients to provide and receive care. Foot/ankle and hand centers are being created as well to provide patients with more comprehensive care.

As you read the following chapters, you will benefit from the cumulative experience of our team and other colleagues who have been involved in the development and management of orthopedic and spine destination centers. Even in today's fast-changing, increasingly technological world, the principles of leadership, excellence, management, patient-centric care, measuring results, and process improvement discussed in the pages that follow will endure.

Endnotes

1. Catherine Arnst, "U.S. Health-Care System Gets a 'D'," *Business Week, www.businessweek.com/technology/content/sep2006/tc20060921_053503.htm* (accessed June 18, 2009).

Defining and Pursuing Excellence

Contributing writers: Judy Jones, MS, David Steele, MD, MBA, Chad McClennan, MBA

> *"If you are going to achieve excellence in big things,*
> *you develop the habit in little matters."*
> —*Colin Powell*

Understanding and implementing the core elements of excellence, both big and little, are the building blocks for any successful service-line strategy. Without this foundation, you cannot expect long-term success. This chapter will explore how the term "excellence" has evolved in the healthcare industry in recent years and provide some thoughts on the core elements of excellence. It will also illustrate how our thinking must change if we are to transform healthcare as well as provide guidance on measuring performance based on internal and external sources.

Why Is Excellence Hard to Define?

People's definition of excellence may vary dramatically depending on their point of view. To illustrate this point when speaking to healthcare professionals, I often refer to an industry outside of healthcare with which we are familiar: the airlines.

If you ask a room full of frequent flyers what defines excellence in the airline industry, their answers generally include on-time departure and arrival, baggage arrival on the same flight, short security lines, helpful flight attendants, and ease of reservations. When the same question is asked of pilots or mechanics, excellence is marked by safe departure and landing, up-to-date equipment, and expert maintenance. They define excellence in technical terms related to safety. Ask this question to the finance people, and excellence becomes defined in terms of efficiency and profitability.

As seen in this example, the perception of excellence varies greatly. Passengers have no way to evaluate the equipment, flight pattern, or maintenance records and can judge the flight only by their experience. The pilots and mechanics have different responsibilities and therefore view excellence differently.

What about healthcare?

What is true in the airlines is also true in healthcare. All stakeholders—consumers, providers, administrators, and payers—define excellence differently.

Consumers

The consumers in healthcare are the patients and their family members. Like airline consumers, they often define excellence by their experience with regard to service. The patient is not able to judge the knowledge and skill of the surgeon, nurses, or physical therapists. Patients and families judge quality and competence by things they can measure—service and long-term results. They may evaluate their experience based on the following:

- Education and preparation

- Pain/nausea kept under control

- Communication with the nurses

- Prompt response to call bell

- Noise levels

- Food

- Transition/discharge process

- Success of surgery

- Return to activities

Providers

Nurses, physicians, and therapists think more like pilots and describe excellence in technical terms. Surgeons define themselves as excellent by their training and skills, their ability to utilize the most relevant technology, and their opinion on the clinical result of the operation. Nurses and physical/occupational therapists determine excellence according to their clinical expertise as well. But these same providers define excellence in others not necessarily based on technical expertise, but in terms of service, such as the following:

- Did the physician or department respond promptly to my request?

- Is the operating room (OR) efficient?

- Do I get the same team for all of my cases?

For nurses, the best doctors are the ones who respond promptly. No matter how smart or qualified the doctor, one who does not respond to calls or requests is not considered excellent. Surgeons often define excellence by their personal efficiency and teams. At a recent national meeting, an orthopedic surgeon presented his tracked OR times for primary joint cases on a graph. You could see his times getting shorter each year, indicating that he was becoming more efficient. Then his times abruptly lengthened. What was the issue? Was he learning a new technique? A new implant? The answer was that his scrub tech had moved. She had been most responsible for his efficiencies.

Another surgeon was particularly angered by the fact that he had a different scrub tech each time he operated. He was unable to change this pattern because the OR leadership was more concerned with overall OR efficiency than his personal efficiency. Frustrated, he went to the hospital CEO with a proposition: If the CEO would accept having a different executive assistant each day, he would accept having different scrub techs in the OR.

Administrators

Managers may be judged excellent in terms of budgets, lower costs, and profitability, putting pressure on them to perform. As administrators tend to hear more about problems than successes, they may also view excellence in terms of the absence of complaints or complications that receive publicity. This can result in conflicting messages about what excellence really is.

Payers

Payers think about excellence in terms of total cost, not point-of-service costs. They often consider repeated incurrence of avoidable costs as signs of incompetence. For this reason, the Centers for Medicare & Medicaid Services (CMS) has decided not to pay for certain complications that occur in hospitals, and other insurance companies are expected to follow suit.

For a musculoskeletal subspecialty center to be successful in the long term, you must strive for excellence from the perspective of all stakeholders—the patient, the staff members, the physicians, the finance department, administration, and payers. It is not an easy task.

Are Centers of Excellence Really Excellent?

The terms "excellence" and, particularly, "center of excellence" have been so abused that the public has become numb to their use.

For example, it's all too common to drive up to a hospital and see a huge banner in front of the facility that says "Orthopedic Center of Excellence." Or you click on a hospital's Web site to find the words "Center of Excellence" emblazoned across the screen.

But when you interview the staff and the administration at these facilities, they reveal that their "center of excellence" is a 42-bed unit on the third floor, which looks like any other hospital floor. Multiple nurses and therapists care for the all the orthopedic patients as well as other surgical and medical patients. Few of the nurses, if any, have specialty training in orthopedics. There is no coordinator, no medical director, and the surgeons each have their own processes of care. They don't know what their allogenic blood transfusion rate is, the average knee flexion and extension in total knee patients, the readmission rate, or their contribution margin. They don't even know the infection rate, except that it is "very good."

The nurses state that the surgeons are excellent and have excellent results. However, no one is collecting outcomes. They do not know the percentage of patients who have been relieved of their preoperative pain. They don't know how many returned to work or their hobbies.

Administration says the nurses are excellent. And yet their patient satisfaction is not in the 90th percentile, their market share is average, their net promoter score is 75, and they have a problem with nurse retention.

This description is indicative of many "centers of excellence" found in hospitals. A recent survey of hospitals revealed that 60% of hospitals claim excellence in six service areas or more. Unfortunately, this self-proclaimed assertion is not necessarily fact-based. But who can argue when there are no criteria?

So why do these institutions call themselves centers of excellence? Because their marketing departments decided it was a great service-line strategy. Their competitors were doing it, so why not? I refer to this move as "painting the shack."

Avoid 'painting the shack'

Most service-line strategies for hospitals in the 1990s revolved around marketing the service line without significantly improving it. As some hospitals have learned the hard way, painting the shack does not affect the things that are truly important, such as:

- Patient experience

- Patient outcomes

- Physician and staff satisfaction

- Market share

- Profitability

The term "excellence" has occasionally even been hijacked by the government. In the 1990s, Medicare wanted to bundle payments. They called it a Center of Excellence (COE) Project for total joints. CMS didn't define excellence. To the average orthopedic surgeon, the program seemed more like a way to reduce costs than to reward excellence. The American Academy of Orthopedic Surgery was cautious of the COE Project for the same reason. I wrote to the academy, hoping it would set the bar and define excellence. This was never done, and the COE Project mysteriously disappeared and the hoopla about it died away.

My desire to define excellence did not disappear. Discussing the topic of excellence with many of my service line colleagues, we came up with criteria that we called the "core elements of excellence." Between 2005 and 2006, I evaluated 100 hospital joint programs against these core elements and reported my findings at the Clinical Orthopedic Research Society meeting in September 2008. Most of the hospitals I'd visited had implemented fewer than 50% of the core elements, even though many claimed excellence. The areas that were most lacking included the following (the full list of core elements is provided in Figure 2.2):

- Effective structure, leadership, and accountability

- Consistent systems and processes

- Patient-reported outcomes

- Managing from metrics

The phrase "center of excellence" had been overused almost to the point of irrelevance. I prefer the term "destination center of superior performance." A destination center attracts patients from a much wider geographical base. To attract customers from a wider area, you will need to be a superior performer and get patients raving about you. To achieve this, you must place a priority on each of the following:

- Focusing on the patient experience throughout the entire continuum of care

- Establishing a culture of performance improvement through the integration of every caregiver that interfaces with the patient

- Collaboration among surgeons, hospital administration, and nursing

- Designating dedicated space and staff members for each service line

- Standardizing and simplifying systems and protocols

- Constant improvement obtained through patient, staff, physician, and administration feedback

- Measuring the results of interventions and benchmarking them against others

Core Elements of Superior Performance

To begin the journey toward superior performance, each subspecialty service line must establish a structure in four key areas: people, structure, processes, and results, as illustrated in Figure 2.1.

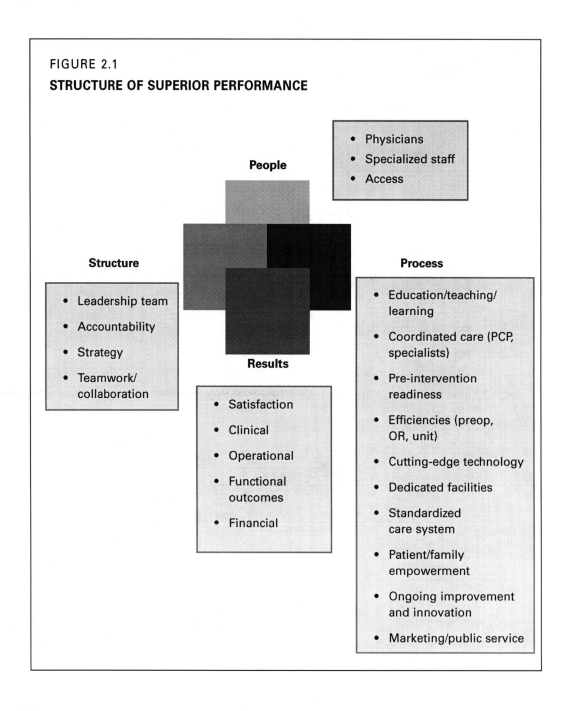

FIGURE 2.1

STRUCTURE OF SUPERIOR PERFORMANCE

People

- Physicians
- Specialized staff
- Access

Structure

- Leadership team
- Accountability
- Strategy
- Teamwork/ collaboration

Process

- Education/teaching/ learning
- Coordinated care (PCP, specialists)
- Pre-intervention readiness
- Efficiencies (preop, OR, unit)
- Cutting-edge technology
- Dedicated facilities
- Standardized care system
- Patient/family empowerment
- Ongoing improvement and innovation
- Marketing/public service

Results

- Satisfaction
- Clinical
- Operational
- Functional outcomes
- Financial

 Orthopedics and Spine

The details of each element in the core areas are further defined in Figure 2.2.

FIGURE 2.2

THE CORE ELEMENTS OF EXCELLENCE

Core element	Definition
STRUCTURE	
Leadership	Formal leadership team, including physician, care coordinator, and administration with authority and accountability.
Strategy	Up-to-date written vision, mission, and philosophy statement. Defined metrics for success.
Performance improvement team	Cross-functional performance team that meets monthly and is dedicated to creating excellent processes, communicating openly, fostering continuous improvement, developing sound long-term strategy, and focusing on timely execution.
PEOPLE	
Surgeon excellence/access	Specialized surgeons who collect outcomes and have implemented a patient-centric care approach.
Primary care involvement	Coordinated approach to assisting primary care providers with becoming an integral part of the patient-centric system of care.
Specialized staff	Specialized staff members with service-specific training and professional certifications.
PROCESSES	
Facilities	Adequate dedicated space to the complete care of the patient.
Superior education	Preparing the patient (and family) for a successful surgery by setting realistic expectations and providing consistent, comprehensive preoperative education and preparation in the specialist's office and hospital.

FIGURE 2.2

THE CORE ELEMENTS OF EXCELLENCE (CONT.)

Core element	Definition
Standardized care system	Implementation of a consistent, standardized, and repeatable evidence-based approach to the delivery of care preoperatively, in the operating room, and postoperatively, using checklists where applicable.
Preoperative process	Integration of consistent preadmission processes, including testing and teaching, and anesthesia review prior to the day of surgery.
Operating room safety and efficiency	Effective use of checklists, SCIP measures, and consistent systems with dedicated anesthesia and staff teams to promote efficiency and safety.
Research/ technology	Effective process for evaluation and adoption of new operative care techniques and technology; involvement in clinical research and/or early adoption of proven advances.
Community service/ marketing	Commitment to public education, prevention, and transparency as an integral aspect of marketing.
Teaching/learning	Culture of continuous learning and improvement recognized by regular case conferences, inservices, standard processes for training, and improvement initiatives.
Performance indicators	Formalized processes for measuring, aggregating, trending, benchmarking, and reporting of key service-line indicators for ongoing improvement initiatives. Sources should include hospital data, outcomes, patient satisfaction, employee/ physician satisfaction, network benchmarks, etc.
RESULTS	
Clinical outcomes	Measurement, aggregation, trending, benchmarking (top 10%), and reporting of all relevant clinical data on a quarterly basis to improve patient outcomes (e.g., allogenic blood transfusions).

 Orthopedics and Spine

FIGURE 2.2

THE CORE ELEMENTS OF EXCELLENCE (CONT.)

Core element	Definition
Operational outcomes	Measurement, aggregation, trending, benchmarking (top 10%), and reporting of all relevant operational data (e.g., length of stay, and discharge disposition).
Financial results	Measurement, aggregation, trending, benchmarking (top 10%), and reporting of all relevant financial data, including costs, profitability, growth, and market share.
Functional outcomes	Collection, trending, benchmarking (top 10%), and reporting of postoperative results using industry-validated surveys.
Patient, physician, staff experience/ satisfaction	Collection, trending, benchmarking (top 10%), and reporting of HCAHPS surveys of patient hospital experience. Obtaining specific and more comprehensive patient feedback across all segments of the continuum of care, not just hospital experience, for purposes of learning and ongoing improvement. Obtaining formal physician and staff feedback on a regular basis.
Awards/recognition	Advanced certification, awards, recognition, or philanthropic success.

Thinking and Acting Differently

The transition of medicine from barbershop bloodletting to a respected profession occurred over many years. Along with it evolved the culture and philosophy of medicine we know today. Although much of this thinking served us well for many years, we must make the following mindset transitions if we are to become excellent:

- Emphasize interdependence over independence

- Consider ourselves members of a professional team rather than professionals on a team

- Emphasize systems performance over individual performance

- Consider the patients, rather than the hospital, as the epicenter of the service line

- Include physicians in our definition of customer

- Encourage specialized care (dedicated caregivers) rather than general care

- Promote professional excellence with less regard to fairness

- Promote value over quality

- Favor real measurements over anecdotal impressions of excellence

 Orthopedics and Spine

Moving away from individualistic thought

At a recent orthopedic conference, I listened to one physician after another provide his or her outstanding results. After being introduced as the final speaker, I said, "We've just heard one doctor after another present outstanding results, but I am here to tell you none of the results were theirs." You could have heard a pin drop. I continued, "You see, the results were not the individual physicians', but those of their teams." After a collective sigh of relief, the crowd acknowledged that what I said was true. None of the results presented could have been accomplished without an effective team doing its job: the internist who prepared the patient for surgery, the nurse who provided preoperative care and education, the OR nurse who administered the antibiotics at just the right time to prevent infection, sterile processing, the anesthesiologist, the scrub tech, the post-anesthesia care unit nurse, the floor nurse, the physical therapist, and so on.

However, this point isn't as obvious as it should be because it goes against the way we are prepared for our careers in healthcare. Most physicians, nurses, and other professionals became successful by being competitive individually. With that, we have become fiercely independent, and yet too often accept accountability for just our little portion of the big picture. As a result, people tend to work within personal, disparate systems, thus inviting tremendous variability. With variability comes decreased effectiveness and higher probability for error.

Medicine today is often "it depends" care. If you get the right surgeon, the right anesthesiologist, the right nurse, and so on, then you will get the right experience and the right result. Unfortunately, the opposite is also true.

Stephen Covey, in his book *Seven Habits of Highly Effective People,* described independence as the middle of three phases of maturity, with the most immature being dependence and the most mature being interdependence. Business schools emphasize team accountability and reward. For example, my son, while working on his MBA, won a contest and a $10,000 prize. I was thinking he won $10,000, but he clarified that his share was $2,500, with the rest divided among the three other team members. When we create interdependence, we leverage our abilities tremendously. Many are smarter than one.

During a recent site visit, I asked members of hospital leadership whether they were more interested in improving individual performance or systems performance. The chief nursing officer quickly responded that most of the hospital's efforts thus far had been geared toward individual performance improvement, such as through individual performance reviews.

Individual performance is important, but it occurs one at a time. Systems improvements work for everyone and can occur hundreds at a time. To create excellence, we not only need to create teamwork and interdependence, but create effective systems as well.

Putting patients at the epicenter

It wasn't that long ago that most births occurred at home and physicians used the patient's home as a hospital. However, with the increase in the complexity and the focus on perfection at all costs, home care disappeared and the hospital became the epicenter of care. Hospitals were built that were cold, unfriendly, and did not

    Orthopedics and Spine

provide an optimal healing environment. Neither patients nor their families were treated as guests or customers.

But with the advent of patient surveys, their voices can now be heard. Hospitals that create optimal healing environments and are passionate about learning from the patient's perspective will succeed.

Physicians as customers and partners

Despite the fact that only physicians can admit patients, physicians have not been traditionally treated by hospitals as customers. And in many cases, hospital-physician tension has been the rule. When newer techniques made outpatient surgery and care a reality, many physicians decided to partner or joint venture with nonhospital organizations that would treat them as a customer and even provide them equity. The coming shortage of specialists will make competition for the best physicians intense. More and more hospitals are now partnering and even employing these quality physicians. In fact, the very successful orthopedic group that I founded was recently purchased by the hospital. I expect this trend to accelerate.

From fairness to excellence

Although physician and staff satisfaction should be a priority, it is dangerous to compromise excellence for fairness. The stakes in healthcare are very high. When people make errors, someone is going to suffer.

However, I've seen hospitals resist creating a center of excellence in orthopedics out of fear that doing so wouldn't be fair to the other specialties. Similarly, hospitals may refuse to provide orthopedic surgeons with the same scrub tech or nurses for every case because of the notion that it's not fair to place the same individuals in the demanding environment of orthopedics day in and day out. But, as explained in Chapter 4, assembling consistent care teams is essential to providing the best possible care for a specific population.

Unless you make sure fairness takes a backseat to excellence, you cannot have a destination center of superior performance.

From quality to value

It seems every hospital vision or mission statement contains the word "quality" somewhere. Few, however, emphasize the word "value," which simply means quality divided by cost.

The concept of value is often misunderstood in healthcare as solely reducing costs, thus risking lower-quality care. But the lack of meaningful measurements and transparency has prevented us from understanding the relationship between quality and cost, leading to a lack of concern about the waste. Much of what we traditionally do may have little or no real value to our patients.

Although the importance of quality should not be diminished, hospitals should create value committees as well. Improving patient satisfaction and patient outcomes while reducing costs will create more value in our healthcare system. We must understand that "value" is not a dirty word and is necessary if we are to achieve excellence.

From generalist to specialist

Many institutions believe that if everyone is a generalist, it will be easier to deploy people where they're needed. Although this mindset may be appropriate in some situations and unavoidable in others, it often undermines excellence. "A nurse is a nurse is a nurse" is like saying "a musician is a musician is a musician." It's just not so. We must understand that focus is one of the ingredients to creating excellence. Violinists don't always make the best pianists. Repetition and practice makes you better. Given the same skills and motivation, specialists can usually outperform generalists in their specific field. They can handle more patients and do it with a smile. It's more difficult to manage the schedule when you have specialists, but it is a step toward excellence.

From anecdotes to measurements

Most physicians do not measure the results of their interventions. Many of our decisions are made with anecdotal evidence only because we haven't taken the time to measure and aggregate our own data. Without such data, it's no wonder that physicians are reluctant to change certain practices. Many hospitals I visit do not even have a good handle on the measurements that are being done, such as allogenic blood transfusion rates.

In President Obama's address to the AMA on June 15, 2009, he declared that we need to change our system from one that pays for activity to one that pays for results. How this plays out will have profound effects.

Owning the Patient Experience

Whenever I meet with hospital leadership, I ask, "How serious are you about the patient experience? Can you give me an illustration of how you have invested in improving the patient experience?"

When I asked these questions recently, the conversation amongst the leadership lasted for at least 20 minutes. Why? They realized they were only giving the patient experience lip service and should have been doing much more, according to their results. Their Hospital Consumer Assessment of Health Providers and Systems (HCAHPS) scores indicated that only 56% of patients who were admitted to their hospital rated the hospital as a 9 or 10 out of 10, and one-third of patients would not commit to recommending the hospital to their friends.

We must face this reality. The institutions designed to care for the sick do not get high marks from half those they are caring for. Supermarkets get better scores than hospitals when asked about satisfaction with the service. This is a real concern as well as a profound opportunity.

Consumers—or patients, in our case—have become increasingly demanding, as they should. With the advent of consumer-directed healthcare and patients footing more of the bill, their expectations increase. Consumers expect the same experience from their healthcare provider as a top online business, retailer, or company that has invested millions and years in perfecting the customer experience.

Another hospital I know was bragging about an HCAHPS net promoter score of 79%. Leadership was delighted that 79% of patients at that hospital would recommend them. They didn't appear to consider the other 21%. Can you imagine if one out of five folks you cared for would never come back or recommend you? How can you be satisfied with that? It's your reputation and brand. And it's not all about achieving great results, which we know cannot be obtained every time. I learned this firsthand as a college student.

My father, also an orthopedic surgeon, took me into the hospital when he was making rounds on his patients. We walked into the room of a patient who was recovering from a postoperative knee infection. This patient's expectation of a rapid recovery and excellent result had been shattered. He then asked my father to step out so he could speak to me privately. I was thinking lawsuit, but what he said astounded me. He praised my father profusely for the way he had cared for him. Someone who had every right to be upset was not only satisfied but delighted with the care he had received. My own 35 years of experience in medicine has borne this out. Yes, the result matters, but so does the experience. A destination center requires that the patient has an outstanding experience. What can you do about creating a better experience?

Other companies and industries are way ahead of healthcare in this arena. To learn from them, we must understand what matters most and least to patients, as a great experience is defined by both. A great experience results in a positive feeling. It is what companies do and don't do that determines how customers feel about their experience.

Above all, remember that the patient experience extends across the entire continuum of care, just as the customer experience extends across all customer touch points along the entirety of the customer lifecycle.

Healthcare institutions begin influencing the patient experience long before the relationship becomes clinical in nature. As business icon Jan Carlzon pointed out in 1987 in *Moments of Truth,* every interaction with a customer provides a company with an opportunity to define itself to its customer, thus influencing how the customer feels about the company and defining the ultimate quality of the customer experience. Carlzon noted that Scandinavian SAS airlines was not a collection of planes, ticketing systems, vehicles, and other assets, but rather a collection of customer interactions that happen thousands of times each day. The underlying assets enable the experience; the customer interactions define the experience. This concept is just as easily applied to healthcare.

Hospital leadership must fully understand what contributes to and detracts from each of the key ingredients of a consistently delivered great experience. Every manufacturer or designer knows that the user of a product or service is the best source for feedback. The patient is the "user" of our service. We must tap into their values and preferences as much as possible. If they are finding our hospital undesirable, our service poor, our communication lacking, we need to find out why. What characteristics of the experience are they expecting, and where are we under-delivering?

HCAHPS surveys are not designed to provide this information for you. They are a barometer, but not enough to understand exactly what patients want. There are several ways to find out what patients in your service line want.

What patients want

Mining for those key customer values can be done in a variety of ways. One is to have patients complete a very focused discharge survey. I say focused because the survey for joint patients is not the same as for spine or sports. Specific questions are asked related to their experience. Room must be left for comments. A tablet or handheld device can be used for electronic collection of results.

With results in hand, identify trends. If you are part of a multihospital user group, you can gather and compare benchmark data by specific subspecialty service line. The advantage of this approach is the ease of obtaining the results and the laser focus of the survey. A problem with this approach is that patients still in the hospital may be reluctant to be completely honest. This survey misses one of the most important parts of the experience, which is the discharge and transition home.

Another approach is to call or send a survey to the patients a week after discharge. This is a bit inconvenient and more difficult to accomplish, but avoids some of the disadvantages previously mentioned. Comments are usually more forthcoming after discharge.

One of the best ways to understand what patients really want is to invite them back with family or their "coaches" a month after their surgery to a patient luncheon. This is most useful with postoperative spine and joint patients who were hospitalized and have lots to comment about. The staff members and physicians must lead this activity. Patients must be given license or even a mandate to share what could be better. We tell them if they don't give us three new ideas, they will have to pay for lunch. This time of exploring what went right and wrong is very helpful in determining what leads to a great experience. Having employees, surgeons, and administration participate in these luncheons allows them to hear firsthand what needs to be fixed.

Patients will explain elements of the experience that we must then translate into improvement efforts. They will express an opinion that we must then translate and analyze to determine the root cause. The cycle is continuous because patients' needs and expectations are ever evolving. We all expect more from the businesses we encounter today than just a few years ago, and patients are no different. Patients are consumers.

In addition, patients appreciate being made part of the solution. Even if their experience wasn't all that it could have been, the negative feelings are modified by our willingness to engage and encourage them to help us. The nurses and staff members get to see the patients recovered. They also get to hear all the great comments, further confirming that what they do makes a difference.

We have found that patients are not dissimilar to customers when dealing with other companies in other industries. Customers have a set of universal needs as well as needs that are situation- or industry-specific. Across industries, customers value accessibility. Accessibility is measured in terms of time on hold, waiting in line, hours of operation, and more. Healthcare is no different. Patients ask: "How long until an appointment is available? Will I be able to see a particular specialist? How long will I need to wait in the office before my scheduled time?"

Within healthcare, customers also place a heightened value on understandable information and empathy. Customers and patients alike certainly value courtesy and professionalism; however, without appropriate levels of product or service knowledge, customers are left unfulfilled in their quest for resolution. Errors erode the quality of the patient experience, so a focus on accuracy must be embedded within any approach to optimize the patient experience. Now that we're firmly within the era of consumer-directed healthcare, focusing on customer needs is the key to differentiation and profit.

Knowing customer needs, preferences, and relative values alone is not good enough. Organizations must organize efforts around those needs and identify the consistent and measurable capabilities that must be incorporated into their day-to-day operations.

The bottom line: The patient experience may have more to do with your success as a hospital than anything else.

Internal Measuring and Managing

As mentioned previously, most self-proclaimed centers of excellence do not collect enough meaningful data to back up that assertion, let alone to use toward performance improvement.

When I ask most hospitals what makes them excellent, I get answers such as, "we have great nurses" or "great surgeons." I find that interesting, and perhaps true, but not convincing. What I should be hearing are figures for how quickly patients return to work and hobbies, and how many are happy with the outcomes of their surgery.

Unfortunately, the following characteristics seem to be more the rule than the exception:

- Many important measures are not aggregated and, therefore, cannot be shared

- Important metrics that are aggregated are not readily available or known by physicians or staff members

- Rarely is one person responsible for the metrics

- Management is siloed into various departments that don't understand the relationships of their actions upon one another

- Low reimbursement, understaffing, or high implant costs are blamed for most problems, even when the numbers are not known

To call ourselves superior performers, we need to measure what matters, aggregate the data, and put one person in charge of managing these metrics. To be useful, data must be easy to understand and accessible to those who need it. We must watch trends and create benchmarks. And most importantly, we must share this information with physicians and staff members who are in a position to help improve upon it.

As noted earlier, blood transfusions represent one area of measures that hospitals rarely track. For example, do you know the cost of a blood transfusion at your service line, who pays for it, or how many you perform? What steps are being taken to reduce transfusions preoperatively, intraoperatively, and postoperatively? If you don't know the answers or whether the information is even collected, you're hardly alone. It's no wonder that the healthcare system is so expensive and that hospitals struggle to make margins.

Managing from metrics

Effectively managing your service line requires not only an investment in developing a comprehensive system of care that engages all the key stakeholders, but also a commitment to continuously tracking, trending, and benchmarking your performance at the service-line level. Outcomes management is an integral component of a destination center and acts as the driver for continuous performance improvement. Managing from metrics often separates the good from the great institutions. To quote Peter Drucker, the man often credited with inventing modern management, "If you can't measure it, you can't manage it."

There are five key categories of measures you should be tracking:

- Patient experience

- Functional outcomes (i.e., postsurgical results)

- Operational data (e.g., average length of stay [ALOS])

- Clinical indicators (e.g., complications, range of motion, and blood transfusion rates)

- Financial data (e.g., contribution margins and market share)

In general, the traditional management model is weak at collecting and aggregating this data into a comprehensive service-line dashboard that can easily be shared and understood.

Patient satisfaction is tracked most consistently, probably because it has become essentially mandated by the government through financial incentives, has benchmarks for comparison, and is understood by most stakeholders. Unfortunately, in many institutions, patient satisfaction scores are not specific enough to lead to significant improvements. They are often used as a grade to compare against other institutions, rather than a tool to continuously improve. This is especially true when a hospital's percentile ranking is already high.

Surprisingly, hospitals often struggle to report service-line data about costs, contribution margin, net margin, and market share. They therefore cannot effectively analyze differences in cost among physicians or other variables that might drive profitability, nor are they comfortable sharing this data with the physicians and staff members who could help make important improvements. Further, without any benchmarking data for comparison, hospitals do not understand how well they are performing. This lack of transparency leads to problems when administration makes statements such as, "We are losing money on joints." Without supporting data or identification of the root causes, physicians assume that the statement must be false or that it's their colleague causing the problem—and trust is eroded.

Operational data such as length of stay (LOS), discharge disposition, volume, and market share is often but not always available. The data is likewise not typically physician-specific. Again, without benchmark data, it is difficult for hospitals to understand whether their ALOS and discharge dispositions are consistent with practices at other institutions. The discrepancies in ALOS for joint replacement patients can vary from a low of 2.5 days to a high of five days. Discharge to home can vary from 10% to 95%.

Clinical data such as complications, range of motion, distance walked, pain, and blood transfusion rates are rarely available. Although the data may be collected at the individual patient level, it is typically not aggregated in a way that can be tracked by the facility or the physician. So if changes to protocols are made, there is no way to know whether changes were beneficial, except by anecdotal means. The only clinical data that is consistently tracked and benchmarked for surgical procedures are process metrics such as use and timing of antibiotics (Surgical Care Improvement Project metrics), done so because the government has mandated or rewarded hospitals for measuring and aggregating such data.

However, with the advances in information technology and increased attention placed on data management, leading institutions are starting to redefine their approach to service-line management by investing in developing service-line-specific dashboards, identifying reliable benchmark comparisons, and sharing their results with a multidisciplinary team responsible and accountable for service-line performance. Electronic dashboards are now available that make it easy to track, trend, and benchmark service-line performance as well as share it with key stakeholders.

Consider the following issues identified and resolved by five hospitals using the same dashboard:

- When one hospital uncovered significant differences in implant costs among five implant vendors, it shared that data with the surgeons to proactively discuss the need for consolidation.

- Another hospital discovered a very high urinary tract infection rate for its joint patients compared to benchmark averages and began drilling down into the root causes.

- A third hospital pinpointed major differences in reimbursement from private payers, including one that was reimbursing significantly less than direct costs. The hospital presented that data during renegotiations.

- A fourth hospital identified a significant variance in average distance walked among its joint patients after surgery, which was adversely affecting ALOS, and tracked the problem back to the differences in treatments used for pain and nausea management.

- A fifth hospital learned it had certain surgeons who were much more likely to discharge patients to skilled nursing or acute rehab, and discussed those findings in an effort to develop a more standardized discharge approach.

All of these examples highlight the value of managing service-line performance with meaningful data and benchmarks as well as the potential effect on performance improvement. Destination centers must create a data-driven culture, institute accountability for performance, and reward service-line managers for achieving superior performance.

The role of patient-reported outcomes

Although tracking the key performance metrics for hospital activities is clearly critical to managing service-line performance, it is still not enough to call yourself a superior performer. To be truly excellent and have the data to back it up, hospitals need to know the degree to which they are meeting their patients' expectations. Patients choose to have an elective surgery with a particular surgeon at a specific hospital because they are seeking an improvement in their quality of life. Therefore, hospitals that want to differentiate themselves and support their claim of excellence must be able to answer questions such as:

- Was the surgery a success?

- To what degree do patients report less pain after surgery?

- Are my patients able to resume activities?

- How fast can my patients return to work?

Functional outcomes data is rarely collected unless it is a part of a clinical trial, and even then the data usually is not shared with patients or referring physicians. But there are some exceptions, such as the Cleveland Clinic, which publishes its patient-reported outcomes in an annual report available to the public.

In the instances that functional outcomes are collected, this data is effectively used for a variety of purposes, including the following:

- **Supporting informed consent discussions with patients.** Sharing outcomes data with patients quantitatively highlights the risks and rewards and potentially reduces malpractice claims.

- **Marketing to prospective patients.** Perhaps as many as 75% of prospective joint replacement patients are excellent candidates for surgery but put it off because they heard of a bad result. Sharing outcomes reduces the information asymmetry between patient and surgeon, lessens the need for second opinions, and should improve surgical volume growth.

- **Sharing with referring primary care physicians (PCP).** PCPs generally believe that the procedures are less successful than they are. For example, one internal medicine physician told me that she thought lumbar fusions were only 25% successful, when the surgeon said it was closer to 80%. But who can argue when there is no data to support either contention? Sharing outcomes results in stronger PCP relationships and improved referral rates.

- **Negotiating with insurers.** Without empirical data to use in negotiations, hospitals and surgeons are left to negotiate against the market average rates. Sharing outcomes during negotiations alters the paradigm and tests whether the insurer truly believes in supporting and rewarding quality.

Surgeons haven't collected outcomes in the past primarily because it was cumbersome and time-consuming, potentially expensive to aggregate, and no one rewarded them for doing so. That is about to change. Simple methods of data collection using handheld devices in the office or online surveys sent via e-mail have been developed. The American Academy of Orthopedic Surgery is looking to develop a joint registry. Pay for performance is gaining momentum and is transitioning toward pay for results.

Using patient-reported outcomes to improve and market your performance is just around the corner. One easy way is to use a handheld digital outcomes collection (DOC) tool in the surgeon's office to collect preoperative baseline scores and postoperative outcomes results. The data is then downloaded to a secured server and aggregated to produce easy-to-read reports. DOC can also be used to capture patient experience metrics and conduct market research.

The Role of Credentialing and Certification

Although no standard definition of healthcare excellence currently exists, some specialty societies and accrediting bodies have developed programs in which service lines can earn a third-party seal of approval.

For example, the American Society for Bariatric Surgery (ASBS) has established a certification program for its specialty. To become certified, hospitals must adhere to the protocols of the organization, and surgeons must complete a specific number of surgical procedures. The result is that insurance companies will contract only with those facilities that have ASBS certification.

A certification system has not yet been created specifically for the treatment of musculoskeletal disease, orthopedics, or spine. However, there are several organizations that provide their own interpretations of excellence and offer corresponding certifications in various areas, including some orthopedic subspecialties.

The Joint Commission

The Joint Commission's Disease-Specific Care Certification program, launched in 2002, is designed to evaluate disease management and chronic care services that are provided by direct care providers such as hospitals, home care, long-term care, ambulatory care facilities, and disease management providers. Organizations may seek certification for clinical programs representing virtually any chronic disease or condition. A list of certified programs includes but is not limited to:

- Cervical spine treatment

- Hip fracture

- Joint replacement

- Lumbar spine treatment

- Trauma

The evaluation and resulting certification decision is based on an assessment of three areas:

- Compliance with consensus-based national standards and safety goals

- Effective use of evidence-based clinical practice guidelines to manage and optimize care

- An organized approach to performance measurement and improvement activities

Disease-specific programs that successfully demonstrate compliance in all three areas are awarded certification for a one-year period. At the end of the first year, the organization is required to attest to its continued compliance with standards and evidence of performance measurement and improvement activities. To maintain certification, the cycle repeats with an on-site review conducted every two years and a biannual submission of an acceptable assessment of compliance by the organization.

UnitedHealthcare

UnitedHealthcare offers the UnitedHealth Premium Designation Program for Orthopaedics and Spine Care. This program identifies orthopedic surgeons and neurosurgeons who meet criteria for quality and efficiency of care in the care of bone, joint, and spine disorders. Further information about the UnitedHealth Premium Surgical Spine Specialty Centers methodology is available on the Web at *www.unitedhealthcareonline.com.*

The Leapfrog Hospital Survey

Leapfrog is another organization that evaluates facilities and establishes parameters for designation of excellence. The organization was established to provide insights for employers as to where to direct patients. The Hospital Survey,

Leapfrog's hallmark public reporting initiative, was launched in 2001. The survey assesses hospital performance based on four quality and safety practices, endorsed by the National Quality Forum (NQF), that are proven to reduce preventable medical mistakes. Leapfrog is helping to create excellence by focusing on specific processes and people. However, its criteria are not service-line specific.

HealthGrades

HealthGrades is a for-profit organization that provides ratings and profiles of hospitals, nursing homes, and physicians to consumers, corporations, health plans, and hospitals. HealthGrades' independent ratings rely on Medicare data submitted by hospitals. Superior ratings are awarded to hospitals that experience fewer complications than would be expected, which does not necessarily reflect superior results from interventions.

Complication rates certainly represent an important aspect of excellence, but it is not the only one. Imagine if the Super Bowl winner were determined by the fewest penalties rather than the most points scored. Further, the fact that HeathGrades only uses Medicare data, that the data must be supplied to Medicare by hospitals, and that you can use the ratings publicly only if you pay a fee has led some healthcare professionals to question the validity of their use in determining excellence.

BlueCross BlueShield

BlueCross BlueShield also offers a credentialing process for its patients, physicians, and hospitals, and recently added spine care to its Blue Distinction Centers array of programs. Find more information about Blue Distinction programs online at *www.bcbs.com/innovations/bluedistinction.*

Medicare

CMS has made stronger attempts to identify and encourage excellence. Recent CMS initiatives include its requirement that all hospitals participate in its HCAHPS program. Medicare also began rewarding physicians who follow and document certain processes in its pay-for-performance initiative.

HCAHPS assessment of patient experience

HCAHPS is a standardized survey instrument and data collection methodology for measuring patients' perceptions of their hospital experience. Although many hospitals already collect information about patient satisfaction for their own use, until HCAHPS, there was no national standard for collecting and publicly reporting information about patients' experiences that allowed valid comparisons to be made across hospitals locally, regionally, or nationally.

Three broad goals have shaped HCAHPS:

- The survey is designed to produce data about patients' perspectives of care that allow objective and meaningful comparisons of hospitals on topics that are important to consumers

- Public reporting of the survey results creates new incentives for hospitals to improve quality of care

- Public reporting serves to enhance public accountability in healthcare by increasing the transparency of the quality of hospital care provided in return for the public investment

With these goals in mind, the HCAHPS project has taken substantial steps to ensure that the survey will be credible, useful, and practical.

HCAHPS content and administration

The HCAHPS survey asks patients 27 questions about their hospital experience, including 18 items about key aspects of the hospital experience (e.g., communication with nurses and doctors, the responsiveness of hospital employees, cleanliness and quietness of the hospital environment, pain management, communication about medicines, discharge information, overall rating of hospital, and recommendation of hospital). The survey also includes four items to direct patients to relevant questions, three to adjust for the mix of patients across hospitals, and two items that support congressionally mandated reports.

The HCAHPS survey measures service from the patient perspective. This is good, but it has its limitations. Hospitals using HCAHPS sample only a small number of the patients treated. Although this may be statistically significant from a grading point of view, it does not provide enough specific information from a service-line perspective. Further, the patients' responses are limited to the questions asked. Insights on how to lead and manage the service line are often not forthcoming from the results of these surveys.

CMS pay for performance

Physicians can now receive bonuses under the pay-for-performance programs. Several of the initiatives relate to orthopedics:

- Screening for fall risk

- Venous thromboembolism prophylaxis

- Timing of antibiotic prophylaxis—ordering physician

- Selection of prophylactic antibiotic—first- or second-generation cephalosporin

- Discontinuation of prophylactic antibiotics

- Osteoporosis: Communication with the physician about managing ongoing care post-fracture

- Osteoporosis: Counseling for vitamin D, calcium intake, and exercise

Summary

Excellence is difficult to define. However, that should not be a reason to omit that process. Please don't just "paint the shack." Don't be like so many other hospitals that advertise excellence before they've created it. Simply creating a subspecialty musculoskeletal service line will not ensure excellence or superior performance. You must at least implement most of the core elements of excellence outlined in this chapter. This requires coordination of many things, including great people, leadership and structure, effective systems, and results that are measured and proven. It is the foundation from which everything else is built.

Begin with the end in mind. To call ourselves superior performers, we need to measure what matters, aggregate the data, and put one person in charge of managing these metrics. To be useful, data must be easy to understand and accessible to those who need it. We must watch trends and benchmark ourselves against others. And most importantly, we need to share this data with physicians and staff members who are in a position to help us improve.

Have an open mind. Challenge some of your long-held beliefs, but never sacrifice your principles of quality, putting the patient first, and doing no harm. Don't just strive to solve yesterday's problems, but focus on creating a culture that is right for tomorrow's challenges.

The Challenge of Implementation

Contributing writer: Matt Reigle, MBA

Service line development is too critical to approach lightly. It must be seen as a key initiative for the hospital, with adequate resources allocated to the effort. Consider the impact a successfully implemented joint replacement program can have on the bottom line. For example, say the hospital performs 400 total joint replacement cases per year and wants to reduce length of stay—a key benefit of creating a destination center—from 4.6 days to three days on average. That's a reduction of 1.6 days per case, or 40 patient days each year. If the average patient day costs the hospital $500, that's a potential cost savings of $320,000 per year. Over five years, that's $1.6 million in total savings, or $1.2 million in net present value!

So if these initiatives are so important and the return so great, why is the effort often halfhearted? Why aren't adequate resources allocated to the project? Why do most hospitals try to jump right to solutions without giving care to the processes?

Most hospitals simply don't understand all the elements necessary for a proper implementation. Take the process for granted, and your end result will fail or be mediocre at best. Take it seriously and your initiative has the best chance at long-term success.

Assemble Your Teams

One of the keys to leading a successful service line implementation is identifying the appropriate people to serve on the project team—or, more appropriately, *teams*—as we'll discuss. If you take nothing else away from this section, remember the word "team." Just as we approach the clinical component with a patient care team, we need to approach program implementations the same way.

All too often, senior management, in trying to ensure that a program has sufficient oversight and direction (i.e., control), assigns responsibility for an initiative to other senior management team members, often at the vice-president (VP) level. The VP then, in an effort to elicit sufficient physician participation, identifies a doctor or group of doctors to work on the project. VPs might also engage other senior or middle management to serve on the oversight committee or leadership team. Frequent meetings take place, and good ideas often result; however, most of those ideas never materialize. Turning those ideas into action is more difficult than most of us recognize.

Although the development of a leadership team is an important and necessary step in the process, it falls short of effectively sustaining change. A more appropriate team management structure must be focused on guiding and overseeing the implementation effort, while also ensuring that the work gets done. During the early stages of the project, I recommend a two-tiered team structure to provide adequate oversight and effective implementation of the project. The two initial teams include:

- The leadership team—focused on program guidance, support, and oversight

- The implementation team—focused on the design and execution of specific program components

The leadership team

The leadership team is composed of key sponsors from administration, nursing, perioperative services, anesthesia, rehab services/physical therapy (PT), as well as surgeons, the care coordinator, and others as appropriate.

The team is responsible for guiding the overall direction of the project. It creates the vision and mission for the initiative, defines project success criteria, guides the implementation team, and provides direction regarding decisions made over the course of the implementation. Selecting the appropriate individuals is critical. Leaders must have the willingness to implement change, the financial commitment to empower change, key staff members who can lead the change, and support from the physicians.

The leadership team should meet every other week during the early stages of the project to:

- Receive updates from implementation leaders and review project progress

- Empower the implementation team to make key decisions and changes to existing systems

- Troubleshoot and resolve problems

- Ensure open and effective communication across departments

- Remove barriers to program implementation

- Identify additional resources as needed and available (e.g., time, funding, and staffing)

The implementation team

The implementation team includes project participants from each of the departments affected by the implementation effort, including the care coordinator, nursing, PT, finance, dietary, marketing, pharmacy, facilities, registration, case management, and quality. Although the composition of this team may be broader than a typical implementation team, each representative plays a key role in the overall patient experience and cumulatively represents hundreds if not thousands of potential patient touch points along the continuum of care.

Working collaboratively, the implementation team is responsible for putting the project plan into action and taking the necessary steps to implement the program. Although the full implementation team can meet once or twice monthly, a core group of project managers and leaders, including nurse management, PT management, and the care coordinator, must meet weekly to develop the infrastructure of the program, communicate efficiently, and build the components of the timeline. This group should be led by a strong project manager to guide the implementation team, keep the project on track, and report all progress, issues, and requests to the leadership team. This position is typically held by the care coordinator, but until he or she is hired, a strong interim project manager should be identified. Other implementation team members should also be engaged as needed to accomplish their respective tasks.

It is important to periodically (perhaps twice monthly) include the medical director in the implementation team meetings to ensure strong surgeon-hospital collaboration. Involvement of the medical director ensures that the surgeons' views and vision are integrated into the program from the onset. Implementation team members are responsible for:

- Launching the new models of care to their respective departments

- Working through implementation issues, including document review

- Developing protocols and daily routines focused on the improvement of patient care

- Modifying schedules, staffing patterns, and care delivery models

- Developing program themes and creating marketing plans

- Analyzing case volumes, financial models, and projections to improve unit profitability

- Executing improvements

The performance improvement team

As the program progresses toward the launch and the key positions are filled (medical director, care coordinator, dedicated nursing/therapy staff, etc.), a system of regular program assessment and evaluation should be developed. At this time, the two teams should evolve into a single performance improvement team (PIT), described further in Chapter 5. The PIT consists of key individuals, including surgeons, unit leadership, nursing, PT, anesthesiology, and so on, and is responsible for the ongoing improvement and management of the program. Although the PIT is formed prior to the official program launch, the team will continue to meet beyond the launch date and serve as the permanent program oversight committee.

Typically, team members are a subset of the leadership and implementation teams described earlier and may include the medical director, care coordinator, anesthesia leader, unit nurse, PT management, finance, marketing, case management, perioperative services, and volunteer management.

The PIT meetings (and program oversight) should be held monthly and led by the medical director, with direct support and assistance from the care coordinator or service line director and an administrative leader. The PIT is responsible for:

- Reviewing scorecard metrics

- Evaluating patient feedback and increasing patient satisfaction

- Improving profitability

- Identifying opportunities for program improvement

- Making revisions to the program as necessary

- Identifying and leading process improvement initiatives

- Identifying opportunities for improved outcomes

Developing a structured approach to program management will ensure a smooth transition from a nonfocused service line to a well-developed destination center of superior performance. It is important to establish structure early in the project timeline to effectively launch the program, generate the momentum necessary to guide the implementation effort, and establish a solid foundation to ensure long-term success. Begin with the end in mind.

Selecting a project manager

From the beginning of the engagement, senior management should designate someone to serve as the project manager (PM). It is preferable that this person have clinical expertise and, if possible, experience in a business setting. Although effective PMs can come from nonclinical ranks, they may struggle with clinical decisions (e.g., order set standardization and education material development) encountered over the course of the engagement.

Additionally, PMs will have to interact with a wide range of clinicians, and nonclinical professionals may lack the credibility to be taken seriously by physicians, nurses, physical therapists, and others. Having the ability to communicate with these experts on a peer-to-peer basis or at least demonstrating a high level of expertise is critical. Working on the front lines is much different than working as a senior manager, and the experience of knowing what will and won't work in a patient setting may turn out to be one of the key drivers of a great program.

Note that I didn't say that management (middle management) experience was a requirement, which is typically the first characteristic executive sponsors seek. A solid, eager nurse who is interested in growing both clinically and within the organization is often the best choice to lead the project.

The PM should be brought on as soon as the project begins, and his or her time should be focused on the project. Where possible, the individual acting as the PM should be the person whom senior management has identified as the manager or coordinator of the program once it launches. This will avoid the time and cost associated with performing a search midway through the project, as well as the effect of potential programmatic change and unrest once the new manager takes over. Keeping the PM on after the project launches will ensure a smooth transition from implementation to launch and will minimize the negative effect of insufficient knowledge transfer.

Finally, the individual should have a basic understanding in the typical software programs (e.g., Excel, Word, and PowerPoint) or have access to assistance. Knowing how to navigate these programs will allow the PM to communicate effectively, organize his or her thoughts in a structured and easily understood manner, and ultimately save time.

To manage the implementation of a large and important service line takes attention to detail and the ability to manage multiple tasks across varying resources.

Although this sounds obvious, many hospital leaders do not recognize how important it is to allocate the appropriate tools (e.g., dedicated computer and desk space) to the PM, who was perhaps a floor nurse the week before, sharing one unit-assigned computer with the other nurses on the floor.

The Four A's of Implementation

When I was the medical director of the Joint Camp at Anne Arundel Medical Center (AAMC) in Annapolis, MD, I hosted hundreds of hospitals from across the world that were interested in seeing our program in action and replicating it.

Visitors had the chance to sit in on a preoperative class, observe group PT, and meet with their peers on the unit. I even wrote and provided a free guide to implementation, outlining each step necessary to launch a successful program. Despite this effort, few of the hospitals that had visited our facility were able to implement a program of their own. In fact, in 2005, I worked with a medical student and asked him to survey hospitals that had visited AAMC in the prior five years to assess the level to which they had implemented a comparable program. I found that fewer than 10% of the hospitals that had visited AAMC had been able to implement some of the most basic program components demonstrated during their visit.

I quickly realized that the primary roadblock to successful service line development was hospitals' lack of implementation expertise. I had always suspected it, and to a certain extent had experienced it, but I hadn't realized how big the issue actually was. Despite having observed a program in action, having a step-by-step written guide, and having my business card and an open line to many members of the team at AAMC, many well-meaning, highly intelligent, and resourceful individuals from hospitals around the world weren't able to build a comparable program.

So what was the problem? Certainly I wasn't more intelligent than the surgeons at the visiting hospitals. Sure, my team at AAMC was great, but were they that much better than the people who had visited? As it turned out, the issue wasn't the people; it was the system, or lack thereof. Successful implementation begins with a structured system and approach to solving business problems. Although essential, a shared vision and good intentions aren't sufficient. Service-line implementation requires a methodology.

I refer to this methodology as the four As: assess, architect, assemble, and assure. Every one of our projects follows this process. It keeps the project on track, with the end goal in mind and following a methodical, process-based approach to problem solution. Each phase builds upon the prior one until there is a fully implemented and thoroughly built solution.

See Figure 3.1 for an illustration of this implementation methodology.

FIGURE 3.1

IMPLEMENTATION METHODOLOGY

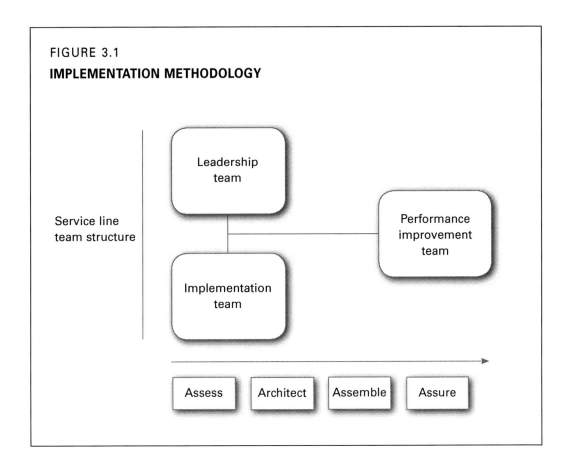

As a surgeon, I can relate to the difficulty healthcare providers may have in adopting this way of thinking. As clinicians, when a life-or-death situation is presented, we quickly make an assessment and act. We don't always have the luxury of time to assess our options, plan our attack, and then carry out a response. But what I didn't realize until I left surgery is that we do subscribe to a structured methodology toward patient care:

- Assess—Ask a lot of questions and diagnose the problem

- Architect—Prescribe a course of treatment

- Assemble—Carry out the treatment

- Assure—Have the patient come back for follow-up appointments

The only difference with service-line implementation is that you are not in an emergent life-or-death situation; use the extra time wisely. Figure 3.2 highlights each of the four As and briefly describes how an effective project team works through each stage. The sections that follow describe each phase in detail, including key questions that must be answered and the primary challenges that must be overcome to manage a successful service-line implementation.

FIGURE 3.2

THE FOUR A'S

Stage	Description
Assess	Each project begins with an assessment of the current situation in order for the project team to understand (1) existing strengths, (2) potential barriers, (3) the magnitude and implications of possible risks, and (4) the feasibility of needed changes.
Architect	The architect phase involves taking the findings from the assess phase and creating a customized timeline that includes the specific tasks needed to complete the project.
Assemble	The building process—implementing changes to processes and systems—takes place during the assemble phase. This continuum ranges from short-term modifications and pilots through all final testing, certification, sign-off, and moves into production.
Assure	The assure phase includes rigorous monitoring of the processes to evaluate performance against goals and act on the resulting insights to continuously improve results.

Assess phase

It's impossible to make a valid recommendation without having some idea of the current state of things at the hospital. What I often find, however, is that the key project sponsors and their leadership team don't know what should be assessed. They know that they have a problem. It could be outmigration, lack of surgeon/administrative collaboration, rising costs, eroding profits, competitive threats, or perhaps all of the above. These are the pain points, the end results, and the key indicators that there is a problem—but not the problem itself. The problem lies within the root cause of each of those pain points, and the assessment should focus on understanding those root causes. Often in healthcare we tend to be "solutioners":

We like to fix problems without going through the rigorous steps necessary to determine their cause.

During an assessment, multiple stakeholders must be interviewed to get a complete view of the initiative's potential and the pending roadblocks. A thorough assessment process takes into account the qualitative points gathered through these discussions and a quantitative analysis of available data to understand the size of the opportunity and/or the resources necessary to make it successful.

Qualitative assessment

The key to leading a successful assessment lies in the questions asked of stakeholders. It is through these question-and-answer sessions that the majority of the insight is gained. The qualitative information obtained may include:

- The size and scale of a problem

- A description of a current process or plans for a new one

- Identification of existing issues and whether current participants want to be part of the solutions

It is important to consider the viewpoints of all stakeholders before undertaking any initiative. Knowing how well and in what manner team members interact with one another helps form a long-term outlook for the service line. Additionally, by asking probing questions, you learn how much ownership each party feels as it relates to the overall patient experience. Figure 3.3 lists some of the key qualitative assessment questions and discussion areas necessary to determine how ready the hospital and key stakeholders are to proceed.

FIGURE 3.3

KEY QUALITATIVE ASSESSMENT QUESTIONS

Stakeholder	Discussion topic
Surgeons	• Physician view of hospital • Current reality in musculoskeletal care • Future goals/fears • Improvement recommendations: patient experience, satisfaction, outcomes • View on hospital-physician collaboration • Needs being met/how they could be better met
Administrators	• Major issues and current approach to address them • Vision/strategic plan for the hospital • Success metrics • Strengths/weaknesses/competitors/brand position • Relationship with surgeons: collaborative or competitive? • Public perceptions: how negative views are being addressed • Hospital-physician goals alignment • PCP loyalty to specialists and hospital • Existing niche service lines/centers of excellence
Anesthesiologists	• Level of engagement/authority/responsibility to the OR • Who selects and reviews performance? • Opinion of the OR? • Level of interaction with the musculoskeletal patient • Issues to be addressed

FIGURE 3.3

KEY QUALITATIVE ASSESSMENT QUESTIONS (CONT.)

Stakeholder	Discussion topic
OR team	• OR effectiveness • Surgeons/leadership opinion of OR • Written vision/mission of the OR • How would you define a successful OR? • Major challenges in the OR • Surgeon/staff interaction • Scorecard: metrics information distribution and utilization
Floor team (PT, nursing, case management, pharmacy, etc.)	• Specialized nursing staff for service lines • Special recognition or training • Surgeon/staff relationship • Staff satisfaction surveys/results/issues • Improvement opportunities
Finance	• Current procedure profitability/reporting process • Level of information sharing with surgeons
Marketing	• Hospital strengths/challenges • Differentiating factor for patients and specialists • Brand message/marketing strategy • Usage of patient satisfaction/outcomes information • Marketing approach: hospital board, PCP, staff, public, prospective surgeons • Level to which surgeons are positioned as experts

 Orthopedics and Spine

Quantitative data

Once it has been established that the key stakeholders are willing to participate and that the service-line focus fits within the hospital's strategic plan, the assessment should turn to a complete evaluation of the numbers to determine whether the initiative is worthwhile. This includes developing a business plan/pro forma, evaluating market share, reviewing case volume and profitability, evaluating key performance metrics, and using a structured approach toward business assessment.

Most finance departments have business plan templates and an established method of projecting success. Despite this, at least 25% of the hospitals I visit have skipped this step and begun an engagement based on gut feelings. Eventually, someone will ask to see the analysis, and it's a tough position to be in if the dollars have already been committed. Take the time to work through the process and meet the hospital's planning requirements. Not only will you have the full support of the board, but you will probably rest more easily at night.

The 'softer side' of the business plan

Nonetheless, my personal experience proves that decisions should not be based solely on numbers. When we launched the joint program at AAMC in 1995, the playing field wasn't level. If I had focused my entire assessment on the quantitative process, we would have never built the program. AAMC is less than 30 miles from Baltimore and Washington, DC. Within 30 minutes of our hospital are some of the most well-respected (if not *the* most well-respected) hospitals in the world. Our market share was low. Outmigration was a huge issue, and no one in his or her right mind thought that a small community hospital would be able to build successful orthopedic service-line programs under those circumstances. Yet my administration had the foresight to consider the softer side of the business plan. The stakeholders recognized a void in the patient experience and believed that by filling it we could differentiate ourselves and build a viable program.

Thirteen years later, I'm proud to say that we did it, and with astounding results. Outmigration is gone. Profitability is up. By the time I retired from surgery in 2006, the joint and spine service lines were the most profitable at the hospital, and market share exceeded the overall hospital market share by more than 40%. Our program has been featured by the Orthopedic Advisory Board, and hundreds of hospitals from around the world have visited us to see the program in action.

The original focus of the program was—and still is—to improve the patient experience (discussed in detail in Chapter 4). Before kicking off the project, we knew that that the financial picture could be positive. But only after assessing the willingness of all key stakeholders to participate and support the program did we know that we had a winner. Limiting your assessment to the financial picture alone may provide you with the size and scope of the potential upside, but only after undergoing a qualitative question-based assessment and asking the tough questions will you know whether your program will become exceptional over a longer period of time.

Architect phase

Would you trust a builder who started knocking down walls and hammering nails without the architectural diagrams? Of course not. Even for small projects around our homes, most of us make a list or draw a diagram before we get started.

 Orthopedics and Spine

Whether we know it or not, we're progressing through the architect phase. Why then do we often bypass this important step at work, when the dollars are big and the impact is even bigger?

Despite its importance, many project teams skip the architect phase and move directly into implementation. Because of the solution-oriented mindset I mentioned previously, it's an easy mistake to make. But we need to resist the urge to jump into a solution without crafting an appropriate plan.

The purpose of the architect phase is to develop the plan, or as I call it, the implementation roadmap (IR), for the team to follow during the assemble phase. Although developing an IR sounds complicated, it doesn't have to be. The key to developing an effective plan is to do it in a way that provides all of the key stakeholders and project team members with an easy-to-understand and descriptive plan for completing the project.

One of the killers of successful implementation is settling for incremental improvements. Without a pressure point, the project often falters. Set a launch date in the architect phase and complete all the items in your plan before that date. An effective IR can range in structure from a simple list of action items with corresponding dates and responsibilities to a more complex diagram or lengthy Microsoft Project Gantt Chart. There are thousands of ways to attack this step; the important thing is that you do it.

Equally important as the list of IR activities is the way the information is presented. By presentation, I don't mean to suggest that the person developing the plan needs to use flashy graphics or the latest tools. Rather, the PM must communicate the content in a way that lets the audience comprehend the information and understand the vision.

Once the content has been presented and comprehended by all the stakeholders, you're ready to proceed to the assemble phase. At times, and specifically for multiphased, complex initiatives, it may be possible to proceed to the assemble phase in parallel with the architect phase. Orthopedic service-line development covers multiple subspecialty areas and may afford you the opportunity to proceed with the implementation of a single-specialty program, such as joint replacement, sports medicine, or spine, while the others progress through the assess and/or architect phase(s).

Assemble phase

During the assemble or "build" phase, changes are made to existing systems, new processes are developed, plans are executed, and structure (e.g., physical space, management structure, and marketing materials) is developed. The assemble phase is typically longer than the prior two phases and requires the most concentrated level of work for the project team.

Unfortunately, because it involves delving into the work and reaping the rewards of accomplishment, the assemble phase is the point at which most hospitals begin. Just like the classic tale of the tortoise and the hare demonstrates, rushing toward a goal without careful planning and purposeful execution will result in ineffective program development and unrealized goals.

 Orthopedics and Spine

The assemble phase should be the easiest to execute. If you've taken the time to thoroughly assess the problem and form an appropriate solution, the implementation should be simple. You know your destination, and you've developed the roadmap; now you just need to follow it. However, it often becomes more difficult than it should be. Unforeseen challenges are encountered, hospital priorities shift, and resistance to change can be powerful. And it's not uncommon for a rogue employee or stakeholder to try to sabotage the initiative. Excuses become commonplace. I'm sure you've all heard one of the following in your hospital:

- "The surgeons won't collaborate with us."

- "But we've always done things this way in the past."

- "There are too many fires to put out. I'll get to it later."

- "But our patients are different."

- "Surgeons will never change."

You must remember that these are normal challenges to any successful project. You've developed the IR to support the effort, and when the challenges present themselves, you should not let any excuse get in your way. Adjust your plan to meet new challenges, but keep your team focused on the goal. As Jim Collins said in his book *Good to Great,* "The enemy of great is good." Don't settle for a good implementation. Focus your team on a great implementation.

Keeping your team on track during the assemble phase requires a disciplined approach toward program development. Many of the keys to success already discussed in this chapter become even more important during the assemble phase. Specifically, make sure you adhere to the following principles:

- **Work the plan.** Remember the phrase "plan the work, work the plan." By now, you've spent many hours analyzing the problems, preparing for change, and developing an IR. Focus your energies on systematically progressing through the work plan. It is always ominous to sit down with a work plan and think, "How will I get all of this done in the time they've given me?" However, if you have carefully and thoughtfully developed a list of key tasks, assigned responsibility to the appropriate people, and accurately judged the amount of time it takes to get something done, you're practically at the finish line. Stick to the plan, hit your dates, and have the confidence that you will accomplish the objective on time.

- **Communicate effectively.** You may have to present ideas and updates in varying forms based on your audience. Focus on what you are presenting and to whom you are presenting. Effective communication doesn't always mean lengthy PowerPoint presentations or e-mail dissertations.

- **Communicate frequently.** By setting up weekly meetings or biweekly project reports, senior management will grow accustomed to the communication plan and refrain from checking in unexpectedly. They will be informed on a regular basis and have the confidence that the progress is being made.

- **Manage issues as they arise.** Don't be afraid of a challenge. If things aren't going as you had planned, or if an unexpected (or expected) issue arises, don't neglect it because you are afraid of the repercussions. Good project managers need to understand that even the best senior executives make mistakes. We're human. But if we address mishaps before they blossom into catastrophes, the project will continue smoothly. Running from issues will only cause them to reemerge later in the project when timelines are tight and budgets are depleted.

- **Celebrate small wins along the way.** The IR gives us a structured map to implementation and a list of near-term deliverables and accomplishments to be celebrated. By acknowledging individuals along the way and recognizing small steps, the project team will remain motivated and excited about completing the project.

- **Delegate.** Just because you have been asked to lead the engagement doesn't mean that you are expected to get all of the work done by yourself. Bring the team of cross-functional experts together and assign tasks and due dates to each of them. Meet regularly as a team and review the progress of each task. Don't be dictatorial in your approach, but do hold people accountable and give them deadlines. If a deadline is missed, before anyone is publicly humiliated, determine whether the overall project deadline will be missed if a task is delayed by a week or two. If the task isn't on the critical path, it may be okay. The person responsible will be grateful that you were willing to work with him or her, and will often perform better and more reliably going forward.

These are but a few of the keys to success during the assemble phase. What is important is to focus on each individual task while not losing sight of the overall objective. Overcommunicate. Keep action lists and update them frequently. Watch deadlines. Progress through the IR purposefully. Work the plan. By following these simple rules, the project will come off on time and on target.

Assure phase

The assure phase begins the day the new service launches and should last as long as the hospital offers musculoskeletal-related services. The focus of this phase is on the continual monitoring, evaluation, and improvement of the program, and is the key to a sustained level of high performance.

Long-term sustainability is possible only through the development of an effective PIT, charged with promoting the cross-departmental communication needed to make substantial performance improvement. For example, the physical therapist needs to talk with the anesthesiologist and explain the effect of postsurgical nausea on patient performance on postop day one. The finance team should share service-line profitability with the physicians and other team members so they can work together to identify ways to improve that profitability. Post-stay, long-term functional outcome data collected in the surgeon's office should be shared with the patient care team in the hospital. Only through the development of an effective PIT can a forum for these discussions be developed. The team must be empowered by senior management to make tough decisions. This can be a huge culture change for many organizations, but in the end, it will pay off.

Effective PITs must make decisions based on data. As such, information from various areas and perhaps disparate systems must be collected, aggregated, and reported on a regular basis. I typically recommend that the care coordinator or service line director, alongside the medical director and an administrative lead, be responsible for preparing the data and sharing it with the rest of the team. When anomalies or problems are identified, the team can collectively discuss the situation and come up with the appropriate response. Mini-projects and/or assignments focused on assessing a particular data point can be given during the monthly meetings, and the results from those assessments can be shared at the next month's meeting alongside recommendations for change. Data collected from financial, operational, clinical, operating room (OR), and patient experience categories should be shared on a single scorecard.

The PIT meetings should also be used to evaluate patient suggestions and complaints. Developing a patient-focused service line requires that their voices be heard. After all, who would disagree that the user of a product or service is the most knowledgeable about how to improve it? When I ran the PIT meetings at AAMC, I would invite a unit-based volunteer to every meeting. This was often the one individual on the unit who made the most personal connection with the patients and was thus able to share specific, actionable ideas for us to make the program better. Including a volunteer in the meetings became a standing requirement for our team that continues to this day.

Although the merits of an effective PIT team are obvious, it is easy to become complacent. You must be vigilant and insist that meetings are held monthly. If team members begin to skip meetings, dismiss them permanently. If the medical director isn't cooperating, replace him or her. If the team members complain that the same issues are coming up over and over again, they aren't doing the things necessary to fix the problems. If you begin to hear that the patients aren't offering any more improvement opportunities when you ask for them, ask again. Even after 10 years of success at AAMC, we still hold patient reunion luncheons every month and ask our patients how we can improve; and every month we get at least three fantastic suggestions.

Don't fall short on your commitment to build a sustainable program. Your investment is too great to let it slide. Don't let the momentum end after the official launch date. If you truly want to build a destination center for great musculoskeletal patient care, make sure to put the structure in place to continually monitor the effectiveness of the program and ensure long-term success.

Keys to Implementation Success

The following rules apply to all four stages of the implementation process and beyond:

- **Don't skimp on planning.** I can't emphasize this enough: Without sufficient attention to the planning phases, the implementation is less likely to succeed. A carefully executed assess phase offers the team the opportunity to evaluate the likelihood for the initiative to be successful and prepare the key players for change. A carefully drawn IR forces the project team to set realistic goals for success, establish expected participation levels, and identify key tasks and timelines for implementation.

- **Engage the physicians.** After careful planning, the next key to service line implementation success is surgeon collaboration. Not engaging surgeons in the process from the get-go is a recipe for failure. Avoid doing it *for* them rather than *with* them. How many times have each of us spent hours crafting the ideal solution, only to have one of the key participants say, "That won't work for me"? I once worked with a hospital in the Midwest that had failed on numerous attempts to change the surgical scheduling process. Each time, it would spend weeks crafting a new solution and preparing to roll it out. And, each time, the solution would be presented to the surgeons (who were employed by the hospital, by the way) only to have them reject the change, or reluctantly agree to it but never follow the new process.

  What did the Midwest hospital do to doom implementation of a new scheduling process? It failed to properly engage its key stakeholders in the design of the program. Had administration gone through even the most basic assessment, asked a few design questions, and made the surgeons feel as though they were part of the process, the initiative would have been successful, and surgical scheduling compliance rates would have been close to 100%.

- **Communicate effectively.** Effective communication accomplishes three key programmatic goals. First, by scheduling regular communication meetings, the project team can keep all stakeholders aware of the project status at all times. This will alleviate the uncertainty that many senior executives have after relinquishing control of an important project. Moreover, by scheduling a specific time and method for project updates, the project team eliminates the need for "fire drills" or out-of-the-blue requests to provide an update. In addition, having a forum for regular communication provides the entire team with a method for making resource requests or proposed changes. In fact, the executive sponsor may be even more likely to grant those requests if he or she feels that the project is being well managed.

Another advantage of effective communication is to mitigate risk and resolve issues. Communicate both the good and the bad—the successes and the challenges—as soon as they arise to minimize the effect later in the project. Perceived failures or approaching difficulties should be presented to the PIT so it can provide assistance.

A clear case of flawed communication occurred at a New England hospital that attempted to build a joint replacement program, hoping to include surgeons from competing practices who were splitting their cases across multiple hospitals. During the assess phase, one of the key drivers of efficiency was a more predictable surgical schedule. Scheduling joint replacement surgeries on specific days of the week would result in a more predictable daily census and allow for resources (e.g., patient rooms and staff members) to be dedicated to the unit.

Unfortunately, the highest-volume surgeon performed cases on the most inefficient day of the week, negating the benefit of changes to the other surgeons' schedules. Rather than approaching the surgeon, discussing the

 Orthopedics and Spine

issue, and engaging him in the solution, the hospital chose to leave the surgical schedule alone. As a result, the hospital never achieved the hoped-for efficiencies. Profitability fell, nurse-to-patient ratios fluctuated, and the joint unit was eventually absorbed back into the general orthopedic unit, increasing length of stay. Ultimately, the high-volume surgeon grew dissatisfied and took all of his cases to the competitor.

What happened here? The leaders failed to attack key issues and address them during the implementation. Small issues grew into larger issues, with their effect being felt in other areas. Investments were lost and the volume went to a competitor—a competitor who didn't have to do anything to win the volume. To make matters worse, the high-volume surgeon who was splitting hospitals had OR time on a better day at the competing hospital. Had my client approached him initially, he may have given up that day at the competing hospital and moved all of his cases to my client on the more desirable day. It's impossible to say what the result would have been had they addressed this issue appropriately.

The third key to good communication is the most obvious. By communicating frequently with everyone on the project team and keeping on top of all of the activities necessary for a successful implementation, the PM will be more likely to lead a successful project. It's important to understand that effective communication does not mean that communication is standardized across all parties. Just as a focus on content and presentation was important during the architect phase, it's equally if not more important during the assemble phase.

- **Appoint a leader.** Successful implementation requires the PM be up to date with the latest project management software packages. This person represents an essential single point of accountability and effective task management. (See Chapter 5 for more about the PM's role.)

- **Get help.** If you don't think your folks have the time, experience, or expertise to develop a destination center with all its elements, then getting some help in architecture and project management from someone who has a solid track record is helpful. Most people hire an architect and a builder when building a house. It certainly saves time, ensures that the house will be built correctly, and quite often saves money.

Summary

As emphasized throughout this book, teamwork is essential to service line success, as is thorough planning. The four A's methodology described in this chapter is one of many approaches to a successful implementation.

Avoid becoming a solutioner. Force yourself and your team to clearly assess the opportunity and ensure buy-in from all key stakeholders. Architect the timelines, resource requirements, and action plans before you begin to do the work. Build the program through key stakeholder input, effective communication, and sound project management principles. Assure long-term program success by establishing the structure for ongoing program evaluation, and arm the team with access to the key performance indicators (financial, operational, clinical, etc.) to make sound business decisions.

4

The Philosophy of Patient-Centric Care

Contributing writers: Judy Jones, MS, Lori Brady, RN, Ron Gaunt, RN

One of the keys to the development of a successful service line is for everyone to agree on the philosophy behind the center. Usually hospitals begin by defining a mission or vision statement and the metrics for success. Of course, these are vital to the measurement of performance. However, it is the philosophy that gives the program its heart and soul. Therefore, the philosophy must be articulated and agreed upon by the surgeons, administrators, and clinical staff. This begins with a short statement that serves as a guide when making future decisions. Keeping to one page, a philosophy statement includes answers to the following important questions:

- Why are we developing the center?

- What are our principles?

- What goals do we hope to achieve?

- How will we function as a team?

The foundation of service line success is a philosophy around the patient-centric model of care. In other words, true centers of excellence look at the continuum of care through the eyes of the patient—not the perception of the hospital or doctor. Many hospitals view the patient experience as an event that begins when patients enter the hospital and ends when they leave. When a patient is successfully discharged, they consider their job done.

That is not how the patient views his or her episode of care, which often begins long before discharge and ends well after. Destination centers of superior performance address the entire experience, illustrated by the patient experience wheel in Figure 4.1.

FIGURE 4.1
PATIENT EXPERIENCE WHEEL

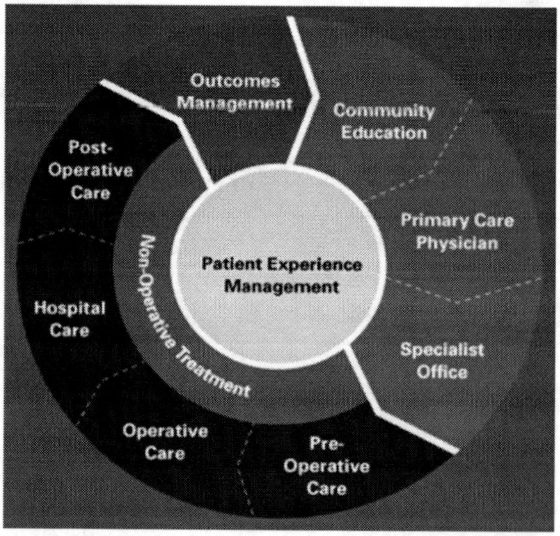

Patients' experiences begin when a problem first arises or comes to their attention as something they should try to prevent. Note that, at this point, a patient may not have even entered the healthcare system.

Community

Thus, patient-centric care begins with a comprehensive community education program and a culture that embraces community service. Each of the subspecialty areas in orthopedics needs to educate the public about the most current knowledge in its particular area. For example:

- In joints, provide advice for managing arthritis

- In foot/ankle, give suggestions to alleviate sore feet

- In sports medicine, offer dos and don'ts for handling injuries on the field

- In fracture care, educate about osteoporosis prevention

- In spine, provide information about nonoperative back care

The goal is to be viewed in the community as the expert. Education will brand the center and establish it as the resource for patients to learn options for treatment. Lectures and seminars provide knowledge and visibility for your surgeons and your clinical staff. Screenings and prevention programs also establish you as a valuable resource.

Your outreach can also extend to fellow professionals and students. For example, spine programs can train school nurses on scoliosis screening.

Sports medicine programs, in particular, always have an element of public service. Offer to provide sports physicals—traditionally held at schools—in your hospital or office. In addition, consider providing an athletic trainer or physician coverage at high-risk sports events in your area.

Primary Care Physicians

When people have pain—back, shoulder, knee, hip—they want relief. They don't think, "My knee hurts; I need joint replacement surgery." Rather, they think, "My knee hurts. I need to know what is wrong and what I can do about it."

The primary care physician (PCP) is usually the first person patients see when they enter the healthcare system to address these issues and myriad others. Thus, PCPs are extremely busy. Explaining all the various options for the treatment of hip, knee, shoulder, or back pain is time-consuming. Your program can help improve patient care by offering help to PCPs.

One technique is to provide educational tools that make it easier for primary physicians to educate patients, such as a brochure listing the top 10 things to do for arthritis. It's also helpful to provide PCPs with a schedule of your upcoming seminars that they can give to patients. Working with your therapists, you can develop arthritis and spine programs—additional services your PCPs should be aware of. Such programs are usually provided by a physical therapist and consist of two

 Orthopedics and Spine

visits: a group session to learn general strategies for managing arthritis or spine problems and an individual physical therapy (PT) consultation. These programs often begin the patient's treatment process.

Many surgeons also provide educational seminars for PCPs to keep them up to date on the latest treatments for knee, shoulder, hip, and back problems. The constant flow of information between the practices is essential for the consistency of care of the individual patient. This is also the opportunity to share your patient-reported results.

By providing educational materials and resources to the PCPs (consistent with the education provided by the specialists and the hospital), you help them do a better job and save time. And you ensure that patients receive a consistent message. Ultimately, you will see those patients who need more complicated treatments.

Above all, make it easy for PCPs to refer patients to the hospital for tests or to specialists for further evaluations. Difficult access can be a major stumbling block that often goes unnoticed until referral patterns have changed.

The Specialist's Office

The next step in the continuum of care is the specialist's office. This is usually the final stop before a patient is scheduled for surgery. Patients must be made to feel that they are in the right specialist's office. If not, they will seek additional opinions and potentially use another hospital.

Create tools and procedures to help with efficiency, patient education, and satisfaction. For example, educate patients immediately as they enter your office with posters and brochures, and include plenty of relevant material in exam rooms as well. Not only will patients learn, but they will perceive a quicker wait time. During the visit, after the physician diagnoses the problem, a patient may be shown videos discussing FAQs before the specialist arrives to close the visit. This saves the specialist time, provides higher-quality information, and gives more opportunity for personal contact with the patient.

At closure, preprinted patient treatment plans can be customized and provided to patients and their families to avoid any confusion as to the diagnosis and recommendations. For patients needing surgery, provide guidebooks that outline preoperative preparation, surgical and hospital expectations, and postoperative care. To avoid confusion, ensure that all material provided to patients is consistent with that given to PCPs.

Presurgical patients will also benefit from access to your outcomes results from similar cases. Of course, you must measure such data first, as discussed in Chapter 2. By sharing this information, patient expectations for the procedure, recovery, and outcomes are properly set.

The navigation and communication from the practices to the hospital (discussed further in Chapter 5) must be easy and clear for patients and office employees. Patients can be introduced to the theme of your program or center (e.g., a spa- or camp-like experience) at the specialist stage as a way to begin building hopeful anticipation rather than dread.

Hospital Preoperative Services

A patient's transition from the surgeon's office to the hospital for testing, education, and the operation must be seamless to ensure the satisfaction of patients and surgeons. Once the surgery is scheduled, the care coordinator—who serves as a patient liaison and advocate—should contact the patient to begin the preadmission testing process as well as the discharge planning process. The care coordinator's role is described further in Chapter 5.

To ensure coordinated, patient-focused preadmission testing and teaching, the anesthesia department should be in charge of preoperative services. Consistent procedures must be established by the program to include completion of the history and physical, testing, risk assessment, family preparation, and any preemptive infection, pain, and nausea control that is planned.

Patient education

Although nurses have typically been in charge of the patient education segment of information delivery, the entire healthcare team—PCPs, specialists, surgeons, therapists, and nurses—has a responsibility to educate and set appropriate expectations for our customers, the patients. The problem is that for many facilities, there is not a cohesive system in place that ensures that patients receive consistent and accurate information regarding their procedure and treatment plan all along the patient pathway. Patients may ask the same question of their surgeon, nurse, and therapist and receive three different answers, which can lead to confusion, frustration, and more calls and questions.

The problem is not a lack of effort or desire to do better, but that a framework is not in place to allow for the coordination and standardization of information. Your approach to information delivery will directly affect the success of your destination center. Information delivery is an all-encompassing term that defines the complete organization of people, processes, and technology used to communicate information to people.

The key lies in the standardization of information delivery. That means the same information is provided and consistent expectations are set for every patient along the entire episode of care. This can be accomplished only with a service-line approach. Our approach provides the necessary framework to make this happen. The entire team is engaged and involved, creating the event that brings together all of the stakeholders to develop the tools and systems needed for effective and consistent patient education and expectation setting. The bottom line: Proper preparation leads to better outcomes.

Operative Care

In many programs, the operating room (OR) functions as its own entity. Service lines must include the OR in their strategic and operational plans. Otherwise, the strategic priorities of the service line will not be reflected in the OR's available time or structure, leading to dissatisfaction among surgeons and patients. Members of the OR, particularly anesthesia, must be part of the team helping patients understand and prepare for their OR experience.

  Orthopedics and Spine

Although safety is a key OR initiative, efficiency is where hospitals struggle the most. Surgeons visit the floor, but the OR is where they live. In essence, the surgeon is your real customer in the OR. The lack of OR efficiency is the most common complaint that surgeons voice. You must incorporate efficiency and the organization's priorities into every center if you are to be successful.

Turn to Chapter 6 for a full discussion about what makes a successful OR.

Hospital Inpatient Floor

Most people dislike staying in a hospital, but it is possible to make the experience positive. There are three elements that make a patient's inpatient stay truly patient-centric:

- Dedicated unit (beds) and staff

- Standardized protocols

- Formal family involvement

Dedicated unit and staff

These are healthy patients who have just had their bad hip or knee repaired. As elective patients, they are expected to participate in their recovery. PT is provided in a group setting. Patients appreciate the camaraderie of being with other patients, and the socialization enhances the recovery process. The space not only includes hospital rooms/beds, but a large space (often called a group therapy room) that can accommodate group PT and luncheons. The space creates differentiation and branding for the service line.

Nurses and therapists must be experts in providing care for these patients. They also become even more valuable to the performance improvement team (described in Chapter 5) when they are knowledgeable about systems and protocols for the specialty. The can identify even subtle changes that affect the patient. This leads to continuous improvement, which is essential in a patient-centric care model.

Consider the typical thoughts of a daughter going to visit her mother in the hospital after total knee replacement surgery:

This place is so busy. I hope Mom is doing okay in here. I wonder if the nurses spend any time with her or explain what will happen next. Hospitals are so noisy—all of the beeps and buzzers and pages. I don't see how anybody could rest in here. And so many people moving so fast in the hallways. They must be in a hurry. Oh, there is the crash cart for emergencies; sure hope they don't need that while Mom is here. Look at that poor person walking around in that drafty gown all by himself. Maybe he doesn't have any family. I've got to be sure I visit Mom every day. I will ask the nurses if I can come in after work—hopefully this won't interfere with the visiting hours or their hospital rules. Well, here is Mom's room; I guess I can just walk in. And there she is, still in bed. Why, her hair isn't even combed.

Many people, including healthcare workers, can probably conjure up a similar experience of visiting a hospital. Hospitals are where sick people go, and the

 Orthopedics and Spine

environment usually reflects the business on hand—but not so with a destination center. Its mission is to establish a culture of wellness for patients, their families, the healthcare providers, and the environment in which they work and recover. The destination center essentially becomes a specialty hospital within a hospital.

The dedicated unit

A dedicated unit is a specific area of the hospital that has separate beds set aside for the care of a particular patient population. Basic elements such as the color of the walls and floor can do much to remove the typical hospital look and feel. Choosing colors and patterns that are warm, updated, and decorative sends the message to the patient that this hospital unit is well maintained, that it is of value to the administration, and that good things must happen here.

Once the aesthetics are defined, the unit must develop its culture. For a dedicated joint unit, items such as wall posters that address FAQs about joint surgery, a bulletin board filled with patient thank-you notes, and a physician and staff "Who's Who" board with team members' pictures help build its personality. Additionally, the unit may have its own signage and a theme, such as nature, hiking, or sailing, featured in the unit's artwork and printed materials. Each of these elements helps brand the center and allows patients to establish a positive relationship with the inpatient environment.

The activity of the unit also helps define its personality. A destination joint center is all about wellness. Patients with a sore hip or knee come to the hospital for joint replacement surgery so they can get back to the business of living life. They are not sick, and we do not want to make them sick by the way we care for them.

Joint patients and their families receive this message in preop class, and it is reinforced by every point of contact along the way, from surgeons to discharge planners. Patients are instructed to bring shorts and T-shirts to wear after surgery and
told that they will be out of bed the same day as surgery or by 7 a.m. the next
morning. They are also told about group PT, which occurs on schedule twice a
day. Families are encouraged to visit the unit at any time and to participate in the
group PT sessions.

Next, let's talk about the patient population of the dedicated unit. It should seem
obvious that a destination joint center takes care of joint replacement patients
and spine takes care of spine patients. This, in turn, means that other orthopedic
patients, general surgery patients, infected patients, and complex medical patients
are assigned to other units. You must establish a clear daily patient routine, an
hour-by-hour outline of patient activity that is directed by nursing and PT plans
of care. In short, nursing and PT must integrate their plans of care to ensure timely delivery of patient care needs and achievement of rehab goals that support the
typical two- to three-day hospital stay. If other patient types—with vastly different
needs—are present on the unit, the joint center staff will be unable to deliver the
care or meet the time demands of this routine.

Dedicated staff

A dedicated staff is a group of staff members selected to provide patient care on
the dedicated unit. Select members demonstrate a positive attitude, clinical excellence, and commitment to maximize the patient experience.

To gain maximum benefit from the dedicated unit, you must staff it with the same set of nurses, assistants, therapists, and even housekeepers and food service personnel. Having a dedicated staff means that each member of the team is knowledgeable about the program, the daily patient routine, the flow of patient activity, and the specific elements that promote a culture of wellness. Each selected team member must be able to demonstrate the right attitude and desire to give 110% to make patients' and their family members' experience the best possible.

I have often heard it said that a "nurse is a nurse." If that is true, then a "doctor is a doctor," too. But in reality, we have family doctors, internists, general surgeons, endocrinologists, neurosurgeons, cardiologists, and even orthopedic surgeons who further subspecialize into sports medicine, ankle, shoulder, and joint replacement surgery. There are countless specialties for doctors; and when you need a specialist, you don't seek the general practitioner.

The same thoughts apply to nursing. All nurses are trained to provide safe and medically sound care. They are taught the basics of all of the body's systems and gain additional knowledge and experience where they work. Employing a dedicated staff on a dedicated unit means that you are providing nurse specialists for this particular patient population. It means giving the nurse the opportunity to move beyond experienced caregiver into expert caregiver. And although experienced nurses are extremely valuable, the art of expertise, of gaining deeper knowledge, can be obtained only through working with the same type of patient day in and day out. One of the nurses I worked with on my dedicated joint and spine center summed it up beautifully. She said, "I have been here two years now, and I can honestly say I know my patients so well that I know what they need before they even ask the question. I have cared for so many joint patients that my ability to anticipate their needs, see trouble coming before it happens, dispel anxiety, and maximize comfort is almost to the level of intuition."

The following three stories illustrate the importance of a dedicated unit and staff.

1. Maryland: Experienced vs. expert/specialty trained staff

It was Wednesday and it seemed quite certain that one of the postop spine patients would not be able to come to the dedicated spine unit. As coordinator for the spine program, this caused me great distress, as I knew the patient's entire hospital experience was at risk by not being assigned to a bed on the dedicated spine unit. I knew I had to do everything I could to meet this patient's needs during his recovery from a multilevel cervical fusion. My first step was to meet with the charge nurse on the med-surg unit. I told her that she would be receiving a postop spine patient who had been to preop class and had certain expectations about pain management, mobility, and prevention of postop complications.

I stayed past my shift to meet with Karen, the evening nurse who would receive the patient from the postanesthesia care unit (PACU), so that I could provide some education about these points. Karen was an experienced med-surg nurse, who listened intently to my teachings and took notes regarding the nuances of managing the patient's postop pain, what do for muscle spasms, how to use position changes and cold therapy to assist with patient comfort, and what to do with the neck brace. I stressed that the patient and his wife, who were both in their 40s, were quite anxious and would do best with a lot of reassurance and explanations of the plan of care. I also told Karen that she and the night shift nurse could call the charge nurse on the spine unit to discuss any questions or concerns about the patient.

  Orthopedics and Spine

The next morning, I went directly to the patient's room expecting to hear a good report. After all, I had educated the nurses and identified people to serve as resources. But I did not get a good report from the patient or his wife. Here is what went wrong:

- **Pain management.** The patient returned from PACU in fair comfort. Within several hours, pain at the incision site and muscle spasms began to set in. The nurse gave the ordered medications, but when they failed to produce relief, took no other measures. The doctor was not called, the pharmacist was not called, and the nurse did not utilize any of the adjunctive comfort measures such as ice, position change, or temporarily loosening the neck brace. The patient suffered needlessly all night. If the patient had come to the spine unit, things would have gone much differently. Here, the dedicated staff knows that securing effective pain management right from the PACU is essential. Once pain control is lost, it is two to three times more difficult to regain. The spine nurses know that if the ordered medications don't work, they must call someone to secure a change in dose or a change in medication. Before I could even ask how the rest of the patient's night was, I had to call the pharmacist to obtain orders for IV medication to bring immediate relief and an order for an appropriate oral pain medication regimen to provide ongoing pain management.

- **Positioning and mobility.** I found the patient sitting in the bed with his knees flexed and his feet pushed up against the footboard. His neck brace was riding up over his chin, and his pillow was too bulky, causing his neck to flex forward. If you aren't comfortable moving spine patients for fear of damaging the surgical site or causing damage to the spinal cord, the prevailing thought is to move the patient as little as possible. In fact, the nurses did not reposition this patient in bed or help him out of bed to walk or stretch his muscles. The patient told me that he got himself out of bed using the rolling over-bed table for support. This news was horrifying. The patient could easily have fallen and damaged the surgical site or caused a new injury. Again, the nurse gave what she knew to be safe postoperative care, but her general knowledge did not enable her to provide the best care for a postoperative spine patient.

- **Family.** The patient's wife was in tears, and all the confidence she had in the hospital, the staff, and her surgeon was quickly eroding. Besides trying to regain comfort for the patient, I had to go into service recovery mode with his wife.

Later that day, the patient was transferred to the dedicated spine unit, where he stayed in the hospital for an extra day to achieve pain control, independent mobility, and patient education, which prepared him for a safe discharge home. The first 24 hours of this patient's hospital stay committed the ultimate sabotage in the spine center's ability to deliver on set expectations and provide the patient and the family member an experience worth promoting.

Karen was a good nurse. She gave good, safe patient care, but in the end was unable to provide the best care possible. Without being part of a spine team and perhaps not seeing this type of patient again for a week or so, it is unlikely she would perform better next time.

2. Oklahoma: The first three weeks on the new destination joint center

Prior to launching the joint center, the orthopedic nurses at his particular hospital would often commiserate with each other about managing postop nausea and vomiting (PONV). Try as they might, no one could put a finger on why this was a problem with some patients and not others. All they knew was that if a patient had this problem, the nurses would be spending the next 48 hours calling the doctor for a variety of new orders. The opening of the joint center, a six-bed, standalone unit, equipped with dedicated nurses, assistants, and therapists, was the critical first step that helped this team get a better understanding of this problem.

Orthopedics and Spine

Because the unit was made up of total joint patients only, the issue of PONV was now readily noticeable, as every patient on the joint unit was having these issues. This meant that the nurses were spending significant amounts of time administering anti-emetics and contacting doctors for new orders, and PT was compromised because patients were too fatigued to come to therapy or ambulate on the unit. All in all, recovery on the joint unit was at a standstill.

Thus, armed with determination and the commitment of the joint center multidisciplinary team, the joint care coordinator and the OR, PACU, and joint center nurses set out to review each patient chart to look for factors that could be responsible for this problem. The chart review proved successful, and the team traced the PONV issue back to the use of a particular anesthetic gas.

This story shows that when a defined patient population is housed on a dedicated unit with dedicated and specialty trained staff members, problems are more quickly identified and owned by a team of individuals committed to resolution.

3. Maryland: Establishment of a stand-alone dedicated spine center

In this story, the hospital maintained a very successful dedicated joint and spine center. As patient populations go, these two patient types work well together, as both usually schedule surgeries in advance, share a focus on mobility, and have a fairly predictable hospital length of stay. As the volumes for each population started to grow beyond the available number of dedicated beds, the spine patients moved to their own unit on a different floor. The spine team knew it would miss the spirit of the combined unit, but was excited for the opportunity to manage its own unit.

Equipped with knowledge and a few tools of the trade, we set up camp and started functioning as a dedicated spine unit. The team's knowledge of the spine patient grew to astounding levels during the next several weeks. I asked myself how this could be. It was the same patients, a subset of the same nurses, the same doctors, and the same plan of care. What could account for this surge in knowledge? Being on our own unit and not having the distraction of joint patients or their separate plan of care allowed staff members to immerse themselves in the needs, discomforts, and concerns of spine patients and their family members. In effect, the accountability for happy and comfortable patients rested on our shoulders. There were no excuses; we owned the patient experience.

One of the newfound discoveries applied to cervical fusion patients. Many cervical fusion patients complain of muscle tightness across the shoulders and a feeling that their arms are heavy and pulling on their neck. This complaint would often persist, even after all available medicines were given and assurances were made that the neck collar was in place correctly and that no obvious postoperative complication was in the making. So when faced with a patient who is uncomfortable, and the usual treatment measures fail to bring relief—and it is just you and your patient—you start trying anything.

I thought back to how I had found relief when I experienced severe neck and muscle spasms, which was to prop my arms up on pillows so that the weight of my arms would not draw heavily upon my neck. Timidly at first, I suggested that we try this position, and within minutes of propping the patient's arms up (full arm support from armpit to fingers), the patient let out a sigh of relief. I was stunned that I had never seen this positioning technique written in any set of postop orders, in my nursing manuals, or mentioned in conversation by the dedicated physical therapist for the spine unit.

This was a great learning experience that occurred because I took ownership of the problem. This was my patient, he was uncomfortable, and I had to do something about it. I was able to apply all of my energy and thought processes to solving this patient care issue. Here is the real key: I was also able to share this information with the entire care team and make it part of our plan of care, not just part of my plan of care.

Standardized protocols

Standardization of care plans, protocols, and orders is an essential part of any service line. The primary reason is that the more variability there is, the more chance there is for error. The philosophy of the patient-centric care model is to eliminate as many errors as possible.

Once in the hospital, the variability in information and expectations only multiplies as more people become involved, including nurses, physical therapists, case managers, and so on. Patients and families may ask the same question of the nurse, surgeon, or therapist, only to get varying answers, wrong answers, or non-answers. For example, a case manager may have to deal with an upset patient and family, even though the patient is doing well and going home, if the expectation set at the office was that the patient would be going to a rehab center.

Within a standardized framework, the entire team is involved, bringing together all of the stakeholders to develop the tools and systems needed for effective and consistent patient education and expectation setting. These include:

- Standardized pre- and postop order sets, which provide the foundation for all of the materials that follow.

- Patient guidebooks distributed to patients at each physician office that contain comprehensive pre- and postoperative instructions, including:

  - Preop conditioning and exercises

  - How to prepare the home for return

- FAQs about the procedure

- What to bring to the hospital, directions, daily routine, etc.

- What to expect after surgery in terms of wound care, medications, pain management, etc.

- Postop exercises

- A diary showing type of surgery and progress

- Group preop classes for patients and families.

- Educational posters displayed on the unit that preemptively answer questions for patients and their families.

- Daily newsletters to keep patients informed of what to expect each day while in the hospital.

- Homework sheets that contain exercises and assignments for patients outside scheduled PT sessions.

- Group discharge classes, which efficiently ensure that patients and families have questions answered prior to leaving the hospital.

- Sets of standardized transition instructions specific to patients going to a skilled nursing facility (SNF), using home health, or headed directly to outpatient PT. Each one of these future caregivers must be given specific instructions.

Formal family involvement

With such short hospital stays today, much of the responsibility that once fell to hospitals is now placed on the family. Despite this, many hospitals still treat family members as visitors—and family members buy into that mentality. This needs to change if we are to ensure that our patients get the best care not only in the hospital, but also when they return home. Although home health is helpful, it can be very expensive and inconsistent. Undoubtedly, insurance companies will eventually bundle payments, as with preoperative care.

Nurses in traditional settings have admitted to me that they dread when families show up. Family members can disrupt the nursing schedule by asking too many questions and, depending upon their personalities, can be quite critical and demanding. Nurses are often grateful if relatives stay out of the way so they can get their work done.

And often, when family members feel in the way, they stay away. In these situations, communication with them about important items, such as discharge plans, is difficult. One of the main reasons that length of stay is often longer than needed is that family members are fearful about taking the patient home or are not prepared to do so. They talk the physician or staff into giving them another day to get ready. This occurs because the family is not usually brought into the care in any formal way.

With the destination center model, we make the family a part of the team with set responsibilities. This engagement ideally begins in the physician's office, but certainly in the preoperative class. We insist that family members attend the class, where their role is formalized, complete with a big "coach" button. Not only is the coach there to encourage and support the patient, but also to learn how to be the chief caregiver once the patient is at home. The coach acts as a second set of eyes and ears at key educational sessions, such as the preop class, exercise sessions, and discharge class.

One of the coaches' responsibilities is to come to postop group therapy classes, where they act as assistant physical therapists. Coaches encourage their loved ones and are shown and taught the dos and don'ts by the physical therapist. Many times, coaches are equipped with digital counters to ensure completion of the activities. If no family member is available, hospital volunteers often take up the coaching role.

One of the responsibilities of the nurse is to teach families the basics of home care. This information is included in a "coach's checklist" used to ensure that discharge medications, wound care, dressing changes, and signs of complications are covered and understood. The coach is expected to sign off on the list before discharge. This greatly reduces the stress on the family at the time of discharge. Coaches also add to the overall patient experience as they interact with other patients and their families, helping to make the hospital stay more enjoyable for all.

Postoperative Care

The episode of care does not end when the hospital stay is complete, but continues to an extended care facility, with home health, or in outpatient PT. Each entity associated with the patient must understand the philosophy of the program and provide the same level of care. To do so, a program must provide the next set of caregivers with all of the communication tools, strategies, and training so that the care progresses seamlessly.

Home health and SNFs

Some patients who have complicated procedures and lack adequate home support must have either home health or be transferred to a SNF. After creating a great hospital experience, one of the most common complaints is that the post-hospital experience did not match the inpatient experience. Home health nurses who don't understand our protocols or don't know what a postoperative wound should look like can spur unhappiness on the part of patient and physician. For example, therapists in the SNF who leave patients in bed most of the day rather than encouraging them to walk around make the patients feel they are regressing, which then becomes a self-fulfilling prophecy, creating frustration and disappointment all around.

Even though we stressed the need for dedicated staff members who understood how to care for these patients in the hospital, we now put them in the hands of caregivers who may not have special experience in dealing with such patients. If we are creating a patient-centric care model, we must take responsibility for educating these folks as well. We need to create specialists in home health and SNFs who understand our program and can maintain it.

One way of doing this is to insist that caregivers spend a day on your specialized unit with your therapists and nurses. Have an educational class for them. Keep a dialogue going between your care coordinator and all outside caregivers and anoint them as part of your team.

Outpatient PT

Once you have a destination center, patients will be coming from farther distances to see you. Putting them in the hands of an unknown physical therapist after surgery can undo much of the great work that was done in the OR and on the floor. Every destination center needs to have a plan to avoid this problem.

Be sure that your patient guidebook has specific guidelines and recommendations regarding PT. When I first wrote our guidebook, I invited 20 PT practices to contribute their ideas, which resulted in a list of nearly 50 exercises. To make the protocol more reasonable, we narrowed it down to the "serious six." With instructions to outside physical therapists on the use of the book, we can eliminate some variation and hopefully any unnecessary risks. Service lines should offer area physical therapists a day on the unit or educational seminars, and physical therapists who don't attend should not be involved in postop care. For distant therapists, Webinars or direct communication with them is another good way to make them part of the team. Remember that your responsibility to patients doesn't end at discharge.

Outcomes Management

The only way a program can continually focus on the patient is through frequent program evaluation, using patient-reported perceptions and collected data to review the clinical, operational, functional, financial, and experience metrics. These metrics become the foundation of the program. Decisions should be made objectively based on the outcomes of the procedure. As discussed in Chapter 2, data must be collected on every patient, aggregated, and presented for evaluation. Changes in clinical protocols, therapy, surgical technique, anesthesia, and so forth can be evaluated to provide the best experience and outcome for the patient.

Summary

The patient does not regard the episode of care based on the hospital stay alone. Rather, treatment of the problem, whether it's knee pain, hip pain, or back pain, can extend over months or even years. Patients have many different encounters, most of them not surgical. A truly integrated destination center provides support to all these potential and real touch points. This coordination instills confidence in patients that the center truly understands their issues and works with all the providers to ensure the best outcome and the best experience.

Five Keys to Structural Success

Contributing writers: Lori Brady, RN, Patrick Vega, MS

A clear and effective structure is essential to service line success. In this chapter, we discuss best practices for creating an effective leadership team, assembling a performance improvement team (PIT), implementing clear systems of care, helping patients navigate, and incorporating teaching and learning into your program.

1. Develop a Winning Leadership Team

Experience has shown that the most effective leadership team consists of a physician service-line director, a nurse, and a product-line manager. Once a leadership team has been developed, its structure must be defined and responsibilities assigned.

Physician leaders

The idea of putting physicians in service-line leadership roles is fairly new among hospitals, but has proven very effective. For example, a recent study conducted by

Kyle Prickett showed that joint programs lacking medical leadership didn't perform nearly as well as those with strong medical directors.[1]

The position of physician medical director may or may not be paid, depending on the size and scope of the service line. Note that these are not the traditional medical directorship roles focused primarily on physician relations. Physician service-line directors, along with the nurse and product line manager, should be responsible for clinical operations, marketing, and financial performance. They provide the vision and strategic planning to accomplish the goals of the service line in alignment with organizational objectives. They serve as a liaison with other physicians, including surgeons, anesthesia, and primary care, to acquire their support in advancing the vision and improving the results of the center.

Many physicians may want the title, perhaps to improve their competitive position, but in reality, few want or are appropriate for the job. The right leader must be respected for good clinical work and perform a significant body of work in the field. The person must be driven to help everyone on your team succeed, and need not be the busiest physician in the organization.

Physicians are experts at diagnosing and solving problems. However, physicians who are too quick to offer their own solutions will stunt the growth of the team. Seek leaders who listen well and will consider the input of the team. Having an attitude of service rather than dictatorship is of enormous benefit.

Select a physician who is passionate about excellent patient care, works well with others, exhibits managerial skills, and sets high standards, especially for him- or

  Orthopedics and Spine

herself. Not every hospital will have such a physician, in which case you'll need to develop one, perhaps by finding him or her a mentor.

On the other hand, codirectorships can be a workable solution for hospitals with several worthy leadership candidates. However, be sure to delineate clearly each codirector's responsibilities.

Sometimes it's clear that only one physician fits the position, in which case an interview process is still necessary to discuss the job expectations, time commitment, and accountability metrics.

Care coordinator

If you don't have a strong clinical program coordinator, you won't have a strong program. This is more of a clinical position than an administrative one, although clinical credentials may not be necessary. This person, often a nurse, will manage all the clinical components of the center and most likely be the face of your program. The care coordinator is the liaison between all the stakeholders that directly or indirectly interface with patients. These stakeholders include physicians (both surgeons and primary care), nurses, physical therapists, discharge planners, quality committees, marketing, and various community resources (e.g., rehabilitation units).

For inpatients, the coordinator will serve as a familiar face throughout the healthcare journey, staying in touch with patients from the time they are scheduled for surgery until several weeks postoperatively, and throughout virtually every step in between. The qualities of an excellent care coordinator are similar to those of the physician, including enthusiasm for adopting a systems approach to care (discussed in the next section), willingness to engage with all stakeholders, and a desire to mentor newcomers.

The care coordinator may report to nursing or hospital leadership, depending on the organization's structure.

Product-line manager

The product-line manager is a lot like a football team's head coach. The head coach takes every piece of information from all assistants and players, synthesizes it, and uses it to make the team better. The head coach is responsible for the wins and losses. He or she reports to the owner, who helps clarify the bigger picture. After several losing seasons, the owner fires the head coach, not the players.

In hospitals, there are managers, finance personnel, marketing departments, nursing departments, operations, and so on. However, often there is no product manager, no head coach who is responsible for every aspect of the product. This responsibility is spread around to many people in their various departments. But with everyone responsible, no one is responsible. No one person has the big picture. Without a head coach, very little changes, despite the good intentions and skill of everyone involved.

The role of product-line manager is typically appropriate for a hospital administrator. As the head coach for the service line, this person will manage the business component of the service line. He or she will be accountable for the patient experience, patient outcomes, and clinical, operational, and financial results of the service line. There may be some overlap with the care coordinator, and in smaller programs (i.e., those with fewer than 500 annual cases), a combination product line/care coordinator position may be filled by one person.

The product line manager usually reports directly to hospital leadership and provides the main administrative support for the program. This person must have significant influence with the executive leadership so that every hospital department, from information technology to dietary, will respond and cooperate when necessary. A good coach will help the team weave through hospital bureaucracy and provide members a realistic sense of where their goals fall within the overall hospital strategy.

Setting expectations

For many hospitals, these three positions that constitute your leadership team may be new positions, and the lines of accountability and authority could be blurred at first. It is important to create, at the very beginning, clear expectations, reporting structures, and accountability. The service-line leadership team must be accountable for all the key measures, such as patient satisfaction, physician and staff satisfaction, volume, market share, profitability, length of stay, complications, clinical results, and more.

All of this data must be collected, extracted, and placed on an executive dashboard. It then needs to be trended against your goals, benchmarked against others, and reported to your PIT. Also ensure that the service-line leadership has a direct reporting line to hospital executive leadership so that key data points may be shared and discussed.

2. The Performance Improvement Team

Most hospitals are structured into clinical silos: physicians, nursing, physical therapy (PT), finance, and so on. Unfortunately, business departments are also often managed independently without much discussion with other departments. Sometimes the leaders of the departments get together, but often they are out of touch with the real issues facing their staff members. Great leadership cannot make up for silo management.

Sometimes called a "quality circle," I recommend service lines assemble a "performance improvement team"—or "PIT crew." No race car driver will succeed without an effective PIT crew, nor will you be able to sustain or improve upon your center without one.

Any personnel—clinical or nonclinical—with the ability to influence the patient experience, patient outcomes, or profitability needs to be on this team. This typically includes not only leadership, but those in the trenches, including joint surgeons; hospitalists; nurses; volunteers; pharmacists; patients; and representatives from the operating room (OR), PT, occupational therapy, anesthesia, case management, finance, marketing, dietary, home health, and extended care facilities. Each of them brings a perspective or solution to issues with which you wrestle. The team should meet regularly, usually monthly, to discuss issues related to the particular service line, whether it's sports, joints, spine, hands, or foot/ankle. The focus of the team should be to improve the patient experience and outcomes while doing it in a cost-effective and profitable way.

                                         Orthopedics and Spine

Getting the team to function like one will require clarity of purpose. I remember reading the story of a janitor at NASA, who when asked what his job was, replied, "Putting a man on the moon." This same common purpose must be understood by all and written down to guide your decisions. Thus, one of your first team activities should be committing your center's philosophy to paper. Similar to the philosophy statement described in Chapter 4, this one-page document should answer the following questions:

- Why are we doing this?

- What is our purpose?

- How should we interact?

- What can everyone expect?

I suggest the leadership take the first crack at writing this statement and then share it with the performance team for additional input. The end product will be a document that gives the group more clarity of purpose. When decisions need to be made, it will be helpful to revisit these words.

Once the PIT crew is in place with its philosophy articulated, maintaining a collaborative culture and making decisions is vital to success. To achieve this, you must:

- Get the right information

- Agree on the facts

- Understand other points of view

Many times, we don't have the right information, or perhaps we think we do but don't agree on the facts. If the facts are in question, ensuing decisions will not be sustained. An appreciation of everyone's point of view is key to creating any working relationship and getting to the best decisions. If people are not talking, don't assume they agree with you. They may feel bullied, intimidated, or frustrated. You must ask PIT members directly for their opinions. The hallway meeting after the meeting is often the undoing of many potential improvements.

PIT responsibilities

The PIT is responsible for the service line in question, not transforming all of healthcare or the entire hospital. As Stephen Covey described in his book *Seven Habits of Highly Effective People,* focusing on your area of concern *and* influence instead of your area of concern where you have no influence is essential. I have been on teams that had such a broad scope that very little was accomplished. The PIT crew needs discipline and focus to succeed.

The following are some helpful hints:

- **Create a "this-is-too-hard box."** Sometimes we get into a situation where the problem is too complicated to solve today or the solution is not obvious. Don't get bogged down in this quicksand. Ask everyone to think about the issue and send you their best thoughts for next month's meeting. Sometimes breaking down the problem into smaller issues helps. As the saying goes, you "eat an elephant a bite at a time."

- **Make some decisions.** Meetings without action become so frustrating we stop attending. Meeting planning needs to occur before the event, with action plans and decisions clearly defined at the conclusion of the meeting. How many times have you witnessed someone start a new topic without having a decision or action plan agreed to on the previous one? Wandering conversations are meeting destroyers. Making decisions and implementing them is the best way to keep the group energized and attending regularly.

- **Get everyone to speak.** Call on the quiet folks—who may be thinking to themselves, "This will never work; they'll see." These silent skeptics often have more ideas than the ones talking; always welcome and require their participation. Remind them that every part of the engine is important if it is to run smoothly or at all.

- **Don't wait for the perfect solution.** Thomas Edison realized it was usually trial and error, not more time or discussion, that led to better solutions. The key here is that you agree that this decision is temporary, and if necessary, it will be modified based on the feedback received.

- **Be considerate about meeting times and locations.** Respect everyone's time and schedule. Surgeons and anesthesia personnel may find it difficult to meet except in the early morning before surgery starts. Consider discussing anesthesia and OR issues first so these folks can get to the OR on time. Some hospital ORs have a later start once or twice a month. Some hospitals don't do joints or spines every day, so off days might work well for meetings. In any event, don't pick a time when people can't meet. Meeting in a conference room on the dedicated floor makes it easier. If that isn't possible, meet in the most convenient place for the physicians. Not every member of the team needs to be present at every meeting or for the entire meeting. Letting physicians know they won't be required will be appreciated, and they will be more likely to be faithful about attending when their presence is needed.

- **Create an agenda that reflects strategic priorities.** One thing that slows improvements is the lack of quality information. Strategic priorities usually include patient/physician/staff feedback, clinical outcomes, and cost effectiveness:

  - *Feedback.* Get feedback from every patient you can. The typical patient satisfaction surveys give you only a high-level view. A destination center must have more specifics on what needs fixing. You can do this with a very specific survey of your own, or consider holding monthly or quarterly patient reunion luncheons to gather this information. Without quality information, you really don't know where the cracks may be.

  - *Clinical outcomes.* Most centers fail to collect or demonstrate data about how well the surgery worked, or things such as blood transfusion rates, etc.

  - *Cost effectiveness.* Quality data showing what and how we are spending combined with quality clinical and satisfaction metrics is essential.

- **Limit hallway fixes.** If you fix it on the fly, usually it doesn't stay fixed or isn't the right fix. Yes, fix it today, but also bring it up for discussion tomorrow. This may enable you to come up with an even better solution

        Orthopedics and Spine

and transfer the information to everyone. Folks are willing to wait if they know their issue is on the agenda and will be addressed.

- **Create a culture of ongoing improvement.** Everyone wants to be on a winning team. Happy patients keep everyone energized, which makes the job more fun. Being on a winning team will help give your center a soul.

It is easier to write about performance than to actually perform. Not every meeting will be great, and not every solution will work. Not every team member will get it. New people will need coaching to understand the culture you have developed. It takes work and commitment. When developing a destination center, this team is usually very visible and highly productive at first. Once the center has been implemented, folks often breathe a sigh of relief that the job has been done and participation lags. This is a red flag. A destination center is perishable, and its work is never done. Improving upon it is the only way to sustain it.

3. Create Consistent Systems of Care

Most hospitals today—whether in the emergency room, the OR, or on the floor—rely on individual performers more than they rely on systems. Although physicians and nurses are by nature intelligent, solid performers, medicine's emphasis on individual contributions has led to some problems.

When each professional works completely alone, there is a significant risk of uncoordinated, linear care. Patients are shuttled from the primary care doctor to the specialist, to the hospital, to the OR, to the floor, and to the outpatient caregivers. Communication is difficult and sometimes lacking. Consistency in message is difficult to sustain. The patient is often left wondering what to do and whom to believe. This current care model is characterized by the three Cs: complex, confusing, and costly.

One of the keys to success is to create systems of care. Systems allow us to create consistency and leverage good ideas over multiple users. Without a system, there is too much variability. Variability leads to inefficiencies and errors. A system will help decrease variability and avoid errors and inefficiencies. A system helps overcome the quality paradox between "first, do no harm" and "to err is human."

From simple to sophisticated

An effective system is consistent, reliable, and reproducible. It does not require one to be a genius to understand it. It is simple enough that it can be used by almost everyone. When you are having a bad day, a system can prevent you from making an error caused by fatigue or preoccupation. A system has backups, and when a system breaks down, it becomes obvious to everyone so that it can be fixed.

Here is an example of an ineffective system: The bathroom door in my office had a little slider. When the slide was pushed one way, it said "vacant," and when pushed the other, it said "occupied." However, it required the user to slide it into the appropriate position. As this door was right near the pod where I was working, I would often see people standing around waiting for the door to open because the sign said "occupied" when it was not. The reason for this is that when people left the bathroom, they were not confronted with the sign or the slider, so they left without sliding the sign back to say "vacant." And of course, users who forgot to slide the sign to "occupied" often found themselves with company.

The error rate on the bathroom door was approximately 50%, which meant it was completely random. Efforts to improve individual performance and behavior through additional training, memos, and so on brought the error rate down to 49%. The lesson here is that attempts to improve performance of a poor system do not work in the long term. Incidentally, the airline industry found a mechanical solution to this problem by linking the bathroom door's lock—needed to keep the door shut and turn the light on—to the vacant/occupied sign on the door.

Another, more complex lesson in systems can be found in the chicken farming industry, which produces a high-value product that is tasty, nutritious, and inexpensive. With this in mind, I decided to visit a chicken farm. In some ways, the thousands of baby chicks running around the farm reminded me of an emergency room on a Friday night in our hospitals.

What I learned was amazing. Farmers have an incredibly sophisticated system for raising chickens, including guidelines on thermostat settings for fans (for both winter and summer), specific migration gestation depending on the number of days, a specific number of hours of darkness and light, the creation of static pressures dependent on the outside temperature, and even a daily mortality record. All of the data was benchmarked against other chicken farmers. My host bragged that she had the lowest mortality record in the entire system. There was more useful data and more consistent systems in the chicken house than I had experienced in our hospital model. This was evidence-based chicken raising. None of the chicken farmers I met were MDs or PhDs, but they all knew their mortality rates and everyone followed a system.

The power of checklists

A checklist is a simple yet powerful system. Dr. Peter Pronovost, a John's Hopkins physician, found that using checklists in the ICU reduced mortality and saved millions of dollars. Dr. Atul Gwande, a Boston surgeon, showed that using a 19-point checklist in surgery preoperatively halved the death rate.[2]

I am often reminded that physicians don't like cookbook medicine. Maybe so, but in one instance they don't mind it: when they get to write the cookbook. Get your physicians together to write the cookbook. In so doing, you will begin to re-create your delivery system and change it from the three Cs (complex, confusing, and costly) to the four Ss: simple, standardized, safe, and with savings. The collection of outcomes, leveraging of knowledge, and standardization of best practices must replace the culture of individual performance, lack of coordination, and slow adoption of change. Future winners will adopt systems of care that allow already outstanding providers to perform even better.

4. Help Patients Navigate

As beneficial as systems can be, sometimes they're not enough to improve care. When consumers seek treatment for musculoskeletal care, it is not uncommon to experience great frustration with all phases of the encounters—access to specialists, referral, treatment, coordination of care, and follow-up. These frustrations arise from common causes:

- Lack of available and accessible information about musculoskeletal problems

- Multiple surgical and nonsurgical providers

- Systems of care that do not communicate with one another and are not clinically coordinated

- Long waits for specialists, particularly spine surgeons and physiatrists

- An absence of readily available information for the patient and family that is helpful in allowing patients to assert a greater role in their care and treatments

This fractured system is not by design; rather, it is the end result of the traditional practice of many specialties and subspecialties that focus heavily on the care they provide. Note that patient and referral source frustrations can arise just as easily from nonclinical interventions (e.g., coordination of consults, diagnostics, scheduling, and communication of demographics information) as they can from clinical interventions.

The dissatisfaction extends to hospitals as well. Frequently, consumers will call what they perceive to be an authoritative resource for all matters medical: their local hospital. Most hospitals have only rudimentary systems for responding and managing individual consumer inquiries. A typical system involves staff members referencing a directory of physicians and offering the caller the phone numbers of one to three physicians that have self-identified as specialists. The caller is then advised to call the offices for scheduling.

Although hospitals are often well-intentioned in this practice, it is generally ineffective and represents a substandard level of customer service. The glaring absence of coordination of access, communication, and service for care seekers is an Achilles heel for hospitals, and particularly spine specialists, in terms of managing the quality of their clinical and business interests.

The navigation model's underlying concepts, processes, and value are designed to address those missing elements. A human touch is also needed to help patients overcome the complexity and confusion often experienced in our healthcare system. As one of my patients remarked, you must find a way to reduce the FUD factor. FUD stands for fear, uncertainty, and doubt. Every patient feels it when entering this foreign environment called healthcare. Helping patients navigate our complex system goes a long way toward reducing the FUD factor.

Although not a new concept, navigation had not been widely used in musculoskeletal care until recently, and it has achieved great success. With an increasing number of patients with no corresponding increase in providers, navigation will play an important role in the future. Navigation, although principally an administrative function in support of clinical services, can significantly influence clinical outcomes such as patient compliance, timeliness, and sequencing of care. Decreasing patient and provider stresses often associated with the process of seeking, receiving, and delivering care will reap enormous benefits. Those hospitals that offer navigation assistance will have an advantage over those that don't. It will be a satisfier for patients, providers, and payers.

To reiterate, the role of navigation is to:

- Reduce the FUD factor

- Coach the patient and referring professional

- Organize key clinical and patient information

- Ensure that all appropriate tests are performed promptly and are available to the specialist

- Be a clearinghouse of key information

- Be a facilitator of communication

The navigation model

Some of the earliest applications of the navigation model first appeared in cancer treatment. Cancer and spine problems, among other disease states, share many challenging care characteristics:

- Typically long and complex treatment cycles

- Numerous surgical and nonsurgical interventions and treatment options for each diagnosis and symptom presentation

- Multiple providers of care

- Labor-intensive administration and scheduling tasks

- Treatment providers spread over multiple offices

See Figure 5.1 for a flow chart illustrating the navigation model.

FIGURE 5.1

NAVIGATION MODEL

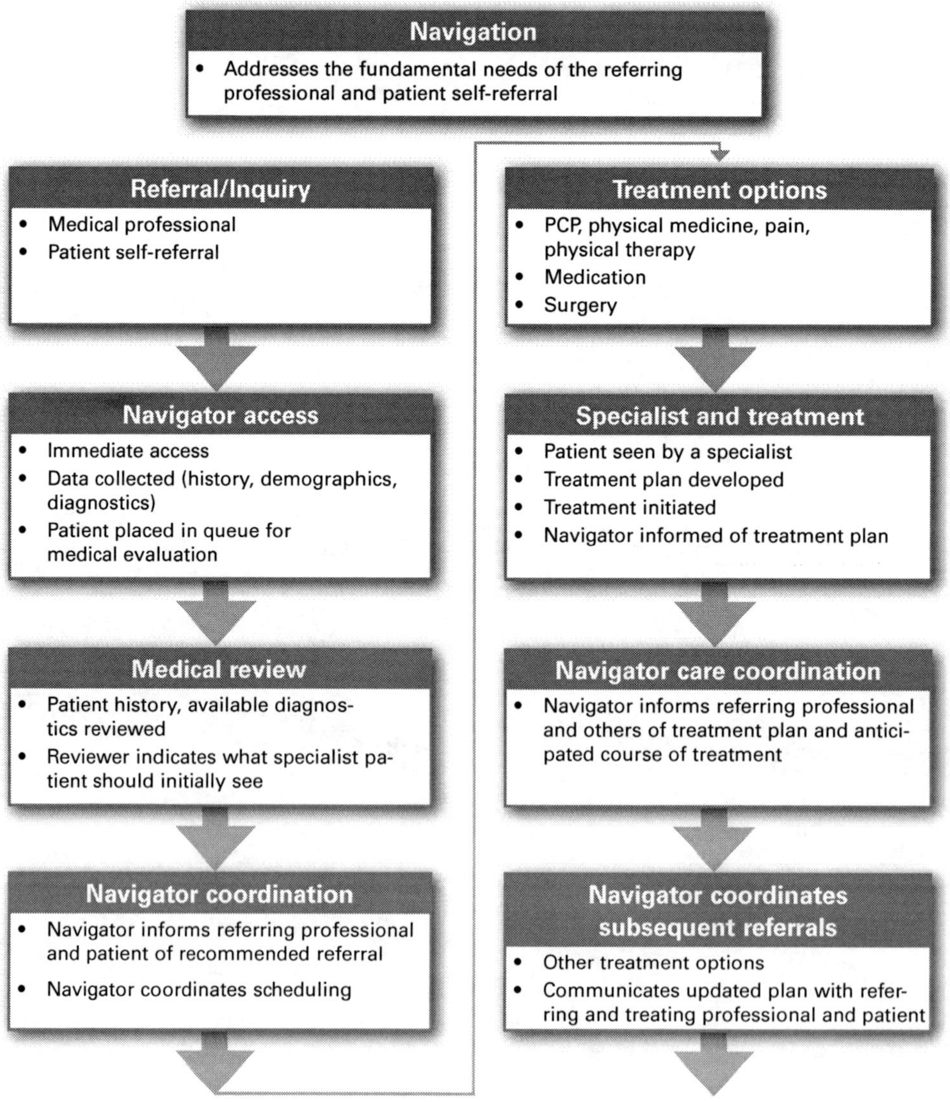

Navigation
- Addresses the fundamental needs of the referring professional and patient self-referral

Referral/Inquiry
- Medical professional
- Patient self-referral

Treatment options
- PCP, physical medicine, pain, physical therapy
- Medication
- Surgery

Navigator access
- Immediate access
- Data collected (history, demographics, diagnostics)
- Patient placed in queue for medical evaluation

Specialist and treatment
- Patient seen by a specialist
- Treatment plan developed
- Treatment initiated
- Navigator informed of treatment plan

Medical review
- Patient history, available diagnostics reviewed
- Reviewer indicates what specialist patient should initially see

Navigator care coordination
- Navigator informs referring professional and others of treatment plan and anticipated course of treatment

Navigator coordination
- Navigator informs referring professional and patient of recommended referral
- Navigator coordinates scheduling

Navigator coordinates subsequent referrals
- Other treatment options
- Communicates updated plan with referring and treating professional and patient

For problems such as back or neck pain, these commonalities too frequently result in long delays in reaching an appropriate professional and treatment modality. One critical difference is the mortality associated with some cancers. In general, the typical spine patient is not at risk of dying but can experience intense discomfort and loss of function.

The goal of navigation is to blend intake, diagnostic, medical, administrative, treatment modalities, and care coordination in an integrated model, not of care, but of care management. When done properly, navigation accrues profound benefits to patients, families, and care providers:

- **For the patient.** Through the use of trained professionals (clinical and non-clinical) communicating a course of care, clinical information, and coordinating scheduling, the patient and family are much more inclined to be prepared for and engaged in their treatments. Patients will have more realistic expectations of treatments, desired outcomes, and options. Patients will also receive rapid access to appropriate care providers. For example, in spine, 85% of patients seeking care for back or neck pain will not be candidates for surgery, but it is not uncommon for patients to be referred by a primary care physician or self-referred to a spine surgeon and endure waits as long as two months, only to be told by a surgeon that theirs is not a surgical condition (either immediately or never) and that they should seek nonsurgical care. Ideally, navigation will identify those clinical and treatment precedents that indicate a path of intervention with a provider most qualified to treat a patient's condition.

- **For the surgeon.** It is not uncommon that surgeons' clinic caseloads are composed of a larger percentage of nonsurgical patients than they prefer. Navigation, by virtue of channeling patients to the most appropriate professional, can result in shorter waits for surgical consults as well as increased surgical yields.

- **For the hospital.** As noted previously, hospitals are often ill prepared to manage self-referred patients seeking care. Ideally, the hospital has invested the correct resources in:

  - Staff members

  - Information technology

  - Well-defined systems

  - Engaging specialists and their respective staff members in a well-defined and broad-based strategy to engage referral sources

  - Exceptional service and communication to patients and referring physicians

  - Hospital-based ancillary services

  - Support of surgery (when indicated) with a comprehensive and remarkable inpatient surgical experience

- **For the payer and care manager.** Navigation should reduce cost by ensuring that the most effective treatments are delivered by the appropriate specialists in an expedited manner. For example, proactive spine professionals,

 Orthopedics and Spine

physicians, rehabilitation facilities, and hospitals will initiate and sustain collection of clinical, financial, satisfaction, and functional data to substantiate the clinical and cost-effectiveness of their care coordination systems and treatment interventions.

Designing navigation

Care providers must first understand how their current systems of clinical and nonclinical interventions function or fail. Additionally, hospitals and specialists must understand and take ownership of the coordination of care that extends beyond their office or hospital walls. They also must take the lead in challenging the status quo to overcome traditional coordination inadequacies.

The primary and support roles for navigation can be filled by clinicians, typically nurses, and nonclinicians. The selection of such will dictate the capabilities of the role. A base expectation is that a navigator will provide care coordination and communication with all stakeholders. Staffing with RNs can provide additional capabilities, such as pretreatment patient education, review of post-treatment questions, and response to treatment.

Software systems have been developed to assist in the navigation process to ensure specialist continuity, patient confidentiality, and coordination of care. These systems were first used in the navigation of spine patients, but recently have been applied to other subspecialties.

For patients and referring physicians, extraordinary loyalty can be fostered through consistent delivery of excellent customer service and coordination of care. The underlying processes of servicing and communicating with all constituents must arise out of a thoughtful redesign of current systems and providers to optimize experiences for all stakeholders.

5. Teaching and Learning

You cannot have a thriving destination center without placing teaching and learning at the core of what you do. Unfortunately, except in academic institutions, this feature is sorely lacking.

The best way to learn is to teach. Most hospitals I've visited do not teach and, therefore, have not become learning organizations. When asked how often they have case conferences, how often the physicians spend time teaching the nurses, or how often they get together to discuss some of the latest thoughts on care, I get blank looks. Most places lack a teaching and learning culture, because no one has organized it. Many get into the habit of just working and then attending or holding a meeting once or twice per year. It is not enough.

Teaching and learning must be built into the very fabric of the service line so that it is regular and relevant. Multidisciplinary case conferences, in which cases are discussed before and after surgery, are at the core of learning. Case conferences should be held monthly if not weekly, particularly in spine.

The benefits are many. First, everyone—from nurses to physicians to patients— learns more. Additionally, these exchanges create a sense of camaraderie among the participants. Physicians who are competitors become collaborators in defining

          Orthopedics and Spine

the best approach to a problem. A greater sense of professionalism and enthusiasm occurs when you are both teaching and learning. Physicians and staff members begin to feel better about themselves and are more satisfied.

Getting started

Getting started is not that difficult. The medical director of the particular service line discusses the concept of case conferences with the team. An appropriate time and format is agreed upon. Invitations are extended. Expectations are set that everyone attending will bring at least one case. In some instances, the physician participation agreement includes language that regular attendance is expected. However, sessions can be videotaped for those who can't make every meeting.

The same is true of nursing inservices. A meeting with the nursing staff may be held to decide on the topics to be discussed. Physicians are assigned to speak on certain topics. The following are some examples of relevant, discussion-oriented topics:

- Current concepts in a particular surgical technique, such as ankle replacement

- Current concepts in managing pain and nausea

- Deep vein thrombosis prevention and recognition

- Blood management

- Infection prevention (including with catheters)

- Fall prevention

- What to do about complaints such as chest discomfort, neck pain, swelling of the feet, light-headedness, or nausea

- How to address hypotension, anemia, hypokalemia, fever, etc.

A 10-question quiz before and after the inservice often helps solidify the information. Continuing education credits usually can be obtained for case conferences and inservices through your hospital education department, as long as the proper paperwork is filed.

The other aspect of being a teaching and learning culture is measuring and aggregating your results. Unfortunately, most institutions measure but do not aggregate their results. They do not know what their allogenic blood transfusion rate is, the percentage of patients with certain pain scores, or what percentage had nausea. The value of this is discussed in the section "Internal Measuring and Managing" in Chapter 2.

The role of research

If you measure and aggregate data, you will become your own research organization. You may or may not choose to publish such data. However, when you are able to show that you can collect and aggregate data, research opportunities with other organizations may be forthcoming, including clinical trials.

The benefits of research are many. First, there is the direct benefit to you and your patients of having access to the latest technology and thinking. Second, being involved in research makes you a better institution, as it forces you to measure,

 Orthopedics and Spine

aggregate, and evaluate. Third, it elevates you in the eyes of the public. Fourth, it can be profitable.

Summary

The triad leadership model is a critical piece in the development of a destination center. The traditional, somewhat passive, medical director role must be replaced by an active, involved, and accountable physician. The care coordinator role must be expanded and strengthened to intersect with many departments. The product-line manager, armed with the data that matters and with the support and advice of the physician and the care coordinator, needs to be accountable for the success and ongoing improvement of the service line.

Leadership can't be successful without an effective PIT crew. This team brings the breadth and depth required to provide the insights that will help leadership make the right decisions. Beware that the PIT is usually the first casualty when a program begins to slide.

Destination centers combine the talents of our healthcare providers with the needs of patients into systems of care. Individual performance is always important, but relying on individuals alone will create inconsistencies and inhibit implementation of new ideas across the entire service line.

Our healthcare system is incredibly complex and confusing. Better systems will help immeasurably and can be incorporated into navigation. Technology and the human touch are both important here. Patients and providers who find navigation difficult will look for alternatives. Navigation must be improved and expanded for inpatient and outpatient care. If we make it easier, we decrease anxiety, improve satisfaction, and improve outcomes. A teaching and learning culture is at the core of excellence.

Quality is cost-effective. The structural components of leadership, PITs, systems, navigation, and teaching will go a long way toward decreasing costs, eliminating redundancy, and improving satisfaction and outcomes.

Endnotes

1. Kyle Prickett and Marshall K. Steele, MD. "Empowering and Mentoring Leadership: The Key to the Implementation of a New Delivery System for Care of Total Joint Patients," Marshall Steele & Associates, *www.marshallsteele.com/articles.asp* (accessed July 16, 2009).

2. Atul Gawande, MD, "The Checklist," *The New Yorker, www.newyorker.com/reporting/2007/12/10/071210fa_fact_gawande* (accessed July 16, 2009).

6

Operating Room Best Practices

Contributing writers: Craig Westling, MS, MPH, Asheesh Gupta, MBA

Every destination center of superior performance has extraordinarily satisfied, loyal patients. The tremendous growth of the programs is largely attributable to word of mouth from satisfied patients. However, let's not lose sight of the fact that surgeons actually bring the patients to the hospital. That's why a key component of our program is to optimize the surgeon experience, which takes place primarily in the operating room (OR).

Generally speaking, the more efficient and productive an OR, the happier the surgeons. Our mantra is to make sure that the surgeons have what they need, when they need it, every time. That requires more than simply having enough of the right instruments and a dedicated, trained OR staff. It also means that cases start on time, rooms are turned over quickly, and productive surgeons are given two rooms as part of their block schedule.

Unfortunately, the strategic priorities of most hospitals do not translate into OR action. Consider a common scenario in which the board approves a strategic initiative to develop a musculoskeletal center of excellence. Although there is much fanfare about hiring new doctors, creating a marketing campaign, and so on, there is too often no plan for:

- Creating more OR capacity for additional musculoskeletal cases

- Increasing the OR budget for more dedicated staff members and/or instrumentation

- Allocating OR time for additional surgeons

Remember, as noted in Chapter 2, a "center of fairness" cannot effectively support a center of excellence.

This chapter contains the key lessons we have learned working in the ORs (and their perioperative support functions) of more than 70 hospitals. When working with clients in the OR, our goals are to:

- Reduce nonproductive surgical time and expenses

- Increase surgeon productivity

- Improve physician and staff satisfaction

Accomplishing these goals supports the case volume growth associated with a successful service line. Simply put, hospitals must streamline their perioperative processes to avoid getting buried by the success of the program.

Key Perioperative Processes

Figure 6.1 indicates the key perioperative processes that contribute to the overall success of the OR.

FIGURE 6.1

KEY PERIOPERATIVE PROCESSES

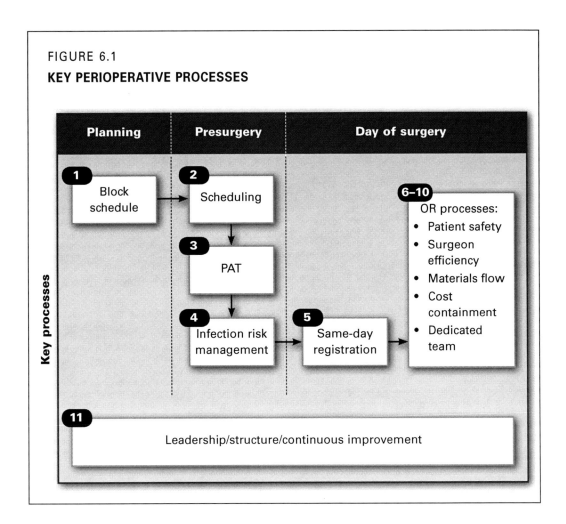

The foundation of the entire model is effective leadership, structure, and continuous improvement. The importance of these three pillars cannot be overemphasized. They are discussed in more detail in section 11, "Governance and performance measurement/improvement."

1. Block optimization

Why it's important

Block allocation and optimization includes (1) the planning process for the management of the OR block schedule and (2) the subsequent matching of resources to support the execution of cases during the block. Block scheduling is your most effective tool for improving the effectiveness and efficiency of the OR.

What we've seen

As mentioned in the introduction to this chapter, the OR schedule must match the strategic priorities of the hospital. We've talked to many surgeons who have said some variation of the following: "I'd love to bring all my cases here, but I can't get them in." The irony is that in almost every instance, the hospital has low utilization and needs these cases. The problem is that other doctors have the ORs locked up, and administration is afraid to take their time away.

The keys to success

We recommend the following actions to optimize your use of blocks:

Orthopedics and Spine

1.1 Block planning:

- Reallocate OR block based on (1) strategic priorities, (2) past performance (utilization, productivity, budget variance), and/or (3) plan of future volumes. Do this at least every other month.

- Conduct quarterly reviews of OR hours vs. plan to allow for a trigger for block adjustments. And really do make the adjustments (don't just threaten).

1.2 Optimize blocks for floor management:

- When making the block schedule, consider how your destination center can be optimally staffed. Predictable surgery days/blocks lead to a balanced census on the inpatient unit, which facilitates efficient staffing.

1.3 Assign double rooms as part of a surgeon's block:

- Assign parallel rooms to productive surgeons as part of their block (rather than as tactical rearrangement on the day of surgery)

- Provide two complete teams (including anesthesiologists), one for each room

1.4 Release block in time to remarket:

- Be proactive with the "remarketing" of released OR time. A block is often released 48–72 hours before surgery, which isn't enough time to get a destination center patient properly prepared (via preop class, performing "prehab," etc.).

1.5 Actively remarket released block time:

- Focus the remarketing efforts to surgeons with case backlogs. The target audience for this remarketing conversation is usually the office manager or the office's scheduling secretary.

- On a weekly basis, let surgeons know about available time during the next eight-week planning horizon.

- Fill the open time on a first-come, first-served basis.

1.6 Report block utilization:

- Make sure the surgeons and OR staff agree on the definition of block utilization. Room time divided by allotted time is a common calculation.

- Communicate this measure and the assignment of block "ownership" to relevant stakeholders (physician group lead or office manager).

- Compute the baseline metric by individual physician (and physician group) for a historical six-month period.

- Set a target (an incremental path to a 75% target utilization is typically achievable).

- Report daily block utilization continuously for a rolling two-week period.

- Review utilization with stakeholders at least quarterly.

1.7 Block management policy:

- The OR block management policy should be documented, including clearly defined measurement and control steps.

- Establish monthly communication between office managers and the OR director. Vehicles for this include:

  - Active strategies, such as a monthly conference call or biannual on-site meeting

  - Passive strategies, such as an OR newsletter or intranet site

2. Scheduling

Why it's important

Scheduling includes the process from (1) the request to (2) reserving a slot to (3) the finalization of the day-of-surgery schedule. A smooth OR booking process includes good communication between the physicians' offices and the OR scheduling function at the hospital. Hospital schedulers should focus primarily on the scheduling of requested cases, whereas the OR scheduling staff should focus on add-ons.

What we've seen

Communication breakdown between these hospital schedulers and office staff members is legendary. Although patients and surgeons simply want to make the appointment and move on, the misunderstandings, frustrations, rework, and overall aggravation for the schedulers is totally unnecessary.

Keys to success

It only takes a few simple steps to straighten out the scheduling process:

2.1 Establish a consistent, efficient case booking process:

- Clearly define the information flow/procedures between hospital OR schedulers and office managers/schedulers

- Use consistent OR booking form types, formats, and submission methods across surgeons' offices (preferably electronic)

- Set up the process so that an OR case posting triggers a notification to preadmission testing (PAT) to contact the patient

2.2 OR time availability:

- The amount of time a patient waits for surgery should be less than one month

2.3 Case sequencing guidelines:

- Define OR schedule sequencing guidelines to enable efficient day-of-surgery flow (considering staff, equipment, and instrumentation resources)

2.4 Communication with patients:

- Once the schedule is finalized, the hospital should manage patient notifications regarding arrival time, as well as any last-minute patient questions

2.5 Freeze the schedule:

- Finalize the surgery schedule by 2 p.m. to enable staff assignments and case-picking activities

2.6 Define a timeline for schedule finalization that allows for:

- Management of add-ons

- Staff assignments by 2 p.m. the day before surgery

- The opportunity for the OR team to review the next day's patient records

- Dialogue between surgeon and anesthesia, if needed

3. Preadmission testing/risk assessment

Why it's important

The purpose of PAT is to perform a risk assessment on each patient to avoid day-of-surgery case cancellations due to preoperative evaluation and testing issues.

What we've seen

Most preadmission preparation processes include primary care physicians and specialists. Too often, the hospital and surgeons' offices are scrambling to track down images, test results, cardiac clearance, etc., the day before surgery. And if there are problems (or charts are incomplete the day of surgery), the case is either delayed or canceled.

Keys to success

The key to a smooth PAT process is to control as many of the variables as possible. Remember, this is a destination center of excellence; you can't leave the proper preop evaluation and management to chance:

3.1 The leader of PAT should be an anesthesiologist:

- Set surgery thresholds, resolve process issues, and communicate changes to the entire anesthesia team

- Define a consistent PAT scheduling process:

  - PAT contacts all surgical patients as soon as surgery is scheduled to direct them toward one of the following paths:

    1. Schedule an appointment

    2. Walk in

    3. Telephone interview only

- Utilize a defined script that includes anesthesia guidelines to assess patients and determine next steps

- Ensure that all required patient tests are performed and information is gathered in one place so an adequate risk assessment can be made three days before surgery

- Send educational packet to patients who do not need to visit PAT

- Ensure PAT involvement begins 15–30 days before surgery (depending on the need for blood management)

3.2 Create a one-stop PAT shop:

- Collect the following patient information during one interaction (the entire process should take less than one hour):

  - Detailed medical and social history

  - Physical exam

  - Required tests per anesthesia guidelines

  - Surgeon-specific testing

  - Education (paper handouts, CD, online information)

  - FAQs (information about pain control, day of surgery expectations, etc.) available in person or via e-mail, phone, or online

- Provide an anesthesia consult if the patient requires/requests one

- Manage blood issues proactively:

  - Do a hemoglobin test 30 days before surgery

  - Correct any anemia prior to surgery

- Reach consensus among the MDAs regarding acceptable risk thresholds for surgery

- Standardize preoperative orders for all surgeons (typically created by anesthesia and approved by surgeons)

4. Preoperative infection risk management
Why it's important
The hospital must have clear strategies to avoid surgical site infections.

What we've seen
The most common patient safety risk is inconsistent processes. Often, this depends on who the surgeon is, so the hospital needs to take ownership and manage the process.

Keys to success
The primary keys to success are comprehensive, consistent patient education and well-defined processes:

4.1 Define a methicillin-resistant *Staphylococcus aureus* (MRSA) strategy:

- A common and effective strategy is to provide nasal Bactroban (mupirocin) three days preop and three days postop

4.2 Provide skincare education at least one week before surgery:

- How to avoid activities that might cause skin abrasions

- Shaving instructions

- Hibiclens (antimicrobial) shower

4.3 Follow your antibiotic protocols, such as:

- Kefzol or derivative within one hour preop

- Restricted use of vancomycin for allergic and MRSA-risk patients

5. Same-day processes

Why it's important

The entire team—including PAT, registration, same-day, and postanesthesia care unit (PACU)—must work well together from (1) initial contact with patients by the PAT to (2) day-of-surgery in processing of patients to (3) actual preparation for surgery and the OR to (4) discharge back to same-day unit or the floor.

What we've seen

A good barometer for the patient experience is to observe the same-day waiting area. How long do patients wait there before they are brought back to a bay? A common reason for long waits is that the same-day unit is understaffed at key points during the day, especially for first cases. This is compounded by the fact that patient charts are often incomplete or tests need to be rerun, causing surgery delays, bottlenecks, and stress.

Keys to success

Processing patients on the day of surgery should be quick, efficient, and patient-friendly:

5.1 Fast-track registration:

- Collect as much information as possible before the patient arrives for surgery:

    - Insurance

    - Copay

    - Past due

    - Advanced directives

- Clearly define and communicate the day-of-surgery admission procedure:

    - Check-in

    - Final patient education

- Provide easy-to-read/follow signage

5.2 Plan ahead for the first case:

- Preassign first cases to a bay the night before

- Escort patients back immediately upon arrival

5.3 Define the patient process:

- OR preparation:

    - Gown

    - IV

    - Preop medications

    - Antibiotics

    - Site preparation

    - Nurse instructs family and patient and sets expectations

    - Surgeon Q&A

    - Anesthesia chart review

    - Anesthesia patient interaction

- Preop goal is a cooperative patient

- Postop goals are pain relief, no nausea/vomiting, and good motor function

5.4 Parallel process as much as possible:

- Use an induction area to begin anesthesia

- Plan activities so that the OR is set up and the patient arrives concurrently

6. Patient safety/experience
Why it's important
Patient safety is paramount.

What we've seen
The most common problems related to safety and experience can be traced to handoffs. Each person who interacts with the patient may not understand how what she or he does fits into the big picture or may expect that others will catch any missed steps. That's not how it works.

Keys to success
Each member of the perioperative team has a role in ensuring the patient's safety:

6.1 Preemptively manage pain and nausea for patients:

- Work with pharmacy, physical therapy, and anesthesia to develop protocols. This is a critical factor in the patient experience, yet anesthesiologists and physical therapists rarely talk to each other about how patients do after surgery.

6.2 Limit traffic in the OR:

- There should be minimal to zero trips in/out of the OR during surgery. Each time the door opens poses an unnecessary risk.

6.3 Prevent blood clots:

- Use foot pumps or sequentials in the OR or PACU

6.4 Eliminate delays from the PACU to the floor:

- Have a dedicated unit for destination center patients

- Coordinate beds to avoid delays in discharging patients from the PACU when clinically ready

7. Surgeon efficiency

Why it's important

Efficient processes mean less surgeon downtime so they can be more productive in the OR.

What we've seen

Just look in any physicians' lounge to find surgeons waiting idly for a room to be ready, or a patient to make it through same-day.

Keys to success

Surgeon efficiency requires a concerted effort by the surgeon, anesthesiologist, and the OR staff:

7.1 Start on time:

- First case should start within five minutes of the scheduled time

7.2 Use double rooms:

- Surgeons who meet the volume and time criteria get two-room blocks

7.3 Establish room turnover targets:

- Agree on a definition of turnover time.

- Set targets for average turnover time, by surgeon. Ideally, daily turnover time targets are set at the morning huddle (given available resources and case details).

- Report actual turnover time to the physician for each of his or her cases at the end of each OR day. This can be achieved with a small whiteboard or log in the scrub area outside the room.

7.4 Use parallel processing to turn rooms over quickly:

- OR circulating nurse notifies the control desk 15 minutes prior to end of case.

- Control desk notifies housekeepers (who have text pagers). Text page at surgery finish so that patient-out-of-room to clean-start time is minimized.

- At room clean completion, housekeeping notifies control desk. Control desk notifies circulating nurse in same-day that patient can be transported.

- Patient is brought to the OR after the setup has started so that the parallel processes will end at the same time and allow for the position and prep activities to start. For example, assume that the room setup time is 30 minutes and the induction time is 20 minutes. The patient should be brought back to the operating room 30 – 20 = 10 minutes after the setup has started (room setup cycle time – induction cycle time in minutes).

8. Instrument/implant/materials flow
Why it's important
Materials management is about ensuring that each surgeon has the right instruments and materials at the right time, as cost-effectively as possible.

What we've seen
You'll be hard pressed to find an angrier person than a surgeon who just broke scrub to go look for an instrument in the central sterile room (CSR) or is told that the screw he needs isn't in the kit or who learns that a tool she uses every time is being used in another room.

Keys to success
A focus on each process is the key to a smooth flow:

8.1 Clearly indicate incomplete cases during the picking process:

- Use a red tag that lists missing items. Eliminate handwritten notes on pick lists. A red tag provides (1) clarity regarding which items are missing and (2) the ability to track items that are consistently missing.

- Have technicians pick the instruments and consumables for a particular case the night before, then document the missing items on the red tag and attach it to the case.

- In the morning, as the case is getting finalized, ensure that the red tag is removed and items that have been cleaned or restocked at night are picked to complete the case. Give the red tag to the OR coordinator or the materials person to refine the pick lists and to verify the par levels for various items.

- Track consistently missing supplies/instruments to determine whether more equipment needs to be purchased or the turnaround process through CSR needs to be refined.

8.2 Avoid flashing:

- Ensure that there are enough instruments to avoid flashing

8.3 Use a visual expediting process in CSR:

- Define work prioritization rules for the prewash queue. This allows the prewash technician to visually identify which load to rinse and load next.

- Use visual designation for trays that require flashing or a quick CSR turn-around (so they can be prioritized by the main central sterile facility).

- Designate a red status for priority work, with red items processed immediately. This means that at the next available moment, the red items are expedited to the front of the prewash queue and then to the front of the washer queue.

- Ensure that the color designation follows the instrument set through the process so the assembly and packing operation can expedite the necessary batches.

 Orthopedics and Spine

8.4 Define a loaner set process:

- All loaner sets should be checked in with a time stamp so that hours prior to surgery can be measured against a recommended policy of loaners on-site no less than 24 hours prior to surgery

- All loaner sets should be reviewed on the decontamination side with a vendor checklist to complete for missing instruments/implants

- Vendor should sign document that indicates sets are clean and complete to the best of his or her knowledge

- A CSR employee should verify the missing parts from the vendor documentation and then cosign to accept the set(s)

8.5 Manage preference cards:

- Clearly define the owner of preference cards

- Update preference cards at least monthly

8.6 Organize instruments/materials:

- Use a case cart system

- Use surgical packs

8.7 Label and store materials:

- Standardize the labeling of carts, bins, and inventory. Each rack, bin, and row should be labeled to allow for easy product picking and efficient put-away strategies.

- Indicate the stocking location on the pick list, rather than just the name and part number of the product.

- Flow rack where possible, where gravity pulls the next item down.

- Use bins for case instrumentation rather than stacking instruments on a cart.

8.8 Promote OR-CSR collaboration:

- Have a weekly rotation of OR technicians through the central sterile department to learn and appreciate the process and instrumentation during the orientation of new staff members

- Have rotating staff identify top three opportunities to simplify trays or improve OR staff members to CSR staff communication

8.9 Provide a clear path for the flow of instrumentation in CSR:

- The workspace should allow a physical flow of instruments for a clear and short path to completion. For example, put the wrapping area adjacent to the assembly area for ease of packing and fewer moves of instrumentation. Move storage racks to allow for a clearly delineated path for the flow of instruments into and out of the autoclave units.

- Designate an area for instrumentation that is waiting to be put away. This area should be minimized so items are stored directly or placed immediately on case carts for the next day's cases.

- In an environment with a high percentage of scheduled cases, the core tech should place instrument sets directly onto case carts for the next day's cases. This eliminates the placement of trays on CSR shelves for six to eight hours prior and the subsequent repicking for the next day's cases.

8.10 Eliminate waste while setting up instrument sets:

- Hold a 30-minute weekly meeting between CSR and the OR coordinator to update the top three pick lists from the previous week. A rotating surgical technician is a valuable resource in this effort.

8.11 Standardize the labeling of wrapped materials:

- Utilize a standard labeling format with set name, surgeon name, and date, written in capital letters

- Use 2-inch wrapping tape for easier labeling

9. Cost containment
Why it's important

Cost containment must be a shared objective of all staff members and surgeons. The entire team should constantly strive to improve processes, make wise purchasing decisions, and be vigilant in containing costs without compromising patient care or safety.

What we've seen

How often has a rep convinced a surgeon to try something new, and then expected the hospital to pay a premium price?

Keys to success

9.1 Demand match:

- Surgeons should always choose the best implant for what is clinically indicated

9.2 Limit vendors:

- Standardize on a limited number of vendors and systems

9.3 Negotiate those implant costs

- Implant cost should be no more than 35%–40% of Medicare revenue if you expect profitability

- Establish rules for the use of off-list implants

9.4 Create a new technology committee:

- Charge this committee to review and decide on surgeon requests for new equipment and other supplies

9.5 Get control over OR inventory:

- OR inventory should be managed by materials management

- OR inventory should be purchased by the purchasing department

10. Dedicated OR team

Why it's important

Having a dedicated OR team for a service line is the single greatest driver of surgeon satisfaction.

What we've seen

Surgeons like predictability in the OR, and when they get new scrub techs every time (or even scrub techs they know but don't like), they get frustrated. However, especially for smaller hospitals, it is not always possible to dedicate teams.

Keys to success

There are a few steps to take to ensure well-functioning teams, regardless of the number of ORs or size of the staff:

10.1 Pick a team leader:

- Establish an OR team leader for the service line

10.2 Dedicate an OR team:

- Train a pool of people who specialize in your service line

- For smaller hospitals, try to always assign an experienced scrub tech to the service line's cases

10.3 Staff appropriately:

- Make sure staffing assignments are aligned with actual block time usage. Aligning with actual vs. planned usage is key, as some surgeons predictably go late every time.

- Underutilization (i.e., running an extra room that isn't fully utilized) is usually better than overutilization due to overtime costs, staff fatigue, etc.

10.4 Have a clear process for day-of-surgery adjustments to staff assignments:

- Designate the control desk supervisor and the anesthesia floor runner to make day-of-surgery adjustments in response to sick calls, case cancellations, case overruns, etc.

11. Governance and performance measurement/improvement
Why it's important

Although each hospital typically has several reports available in its information system and from the manual capture of information, usually the data is not analyzed or reviewed in a manner that guides organizational process management through the achievement of key organizational performance results.

What we've seen

Do you know what critical measures are tracked in the OR? Are those measures and their associated goals shared widely with all staff members and physicians? Do you know how much progress is being made? Are there plans to achieve the goals that aren't being met? Very few people will answer yes to all of these questions.

Keys to success

11.1 OR governance:

- A strong OR committee should be responsible for OR performance and improvement

- There must be evidence of action to achieve established goals

11.2 Perioperative scorecard:

- Use performance measures to create and balance value for patients, surgeons, and staff members.

- Identify a process to select the measures. Include discussions with staff members and physician partners.

- Align performance measures with the needs of all stakeholders. For example, if the physician satisfaction survey indicates that room turnaround time and on-time start percentage are key measures, then those measures must be populated with targets and baselines.

- Have written documentation regarding the formula for calculating each of the measures.

- Share the performance measures with staff members and ask for their input.

- Create a well-deployed operating plan that includes the key performance measures and targets.

11.3 Physician scorecard:

- Determine the top five to 10 measures per surgeon for a monthly report. For example, first case on-time in-room, turnover time, infection rates, OR utilization, cost per case. This is an activity best pursued in conjunction with physician office managers and physicians.

- Consider the "partnering" nature of an OR case to include surgeon/anesthesiologist pairing in the reporting of some key metrics, such as first case on-time in-room, room turnover time, and case duration.

11.4 Surgical Care Improvement Project (SCIP) measures:

- Track and report SCIP measures to staff members and surgeons

11.5 Capture issues:

- Create a process for noting that a service failure occurred and for either (1) stopping to correct the problem (e.g., adjusting a preference card) or (2) communicating in a formal manner the issue to a supervisor or responsible party.

- Document issues (e.g., service failures, incompleteness, or errors).

- Specify issue categories (e.g., patient flow, material shortage, instrument-related, surgeon or anesthesia availability or equipment failure).

- Create a formal mechanism to hear key issues raised by the OR staff. For example, create a "quality circle" to hear the top three issues on a weekly basis.

11.6 Action on issues:

- Fight the war of perception with weekly issue-resolution meetings.

- Track and manage resolution of identified issues with specific action plans, responsibility, and reporting that creates accountability. Report the results (both costs and benefits).

- Show evidence that key indicators are tracked and improved over time. For example, a policy may state that items in red will have a 90-day action plan, so there should be evidence of action plans.

- Have a systematic approach for the creation of action plans:

  - The necessary education and tools should be provided to the action plan stakeholders

  - The deployment of action plans should address the top three issues (at least) per month

11.7 Implement and use a change methodology

- Communicate a weekly change-opportunity list

- Institute change-opportunity execution as part of staff downtime activity

Summary

A well-run, efficient OR is a fundamental element of a successful destination center. The OR must be integrated into the center and reflect the priorities of the organization. There are many barriers to success, not least of which is that hospital leadership doesn't always understand how ORs function. Administrators rarely visit the OR because it requires getting undressed and dressed. As a result, many facilities leave the OR on its own.

The problem with that approach, of course, is that every hospital is competing for excellent surgeons. And because those surgeons spend more time in the OR than anywhere else in the hospital, they need to be viewed and treated as valued customers.

The major complaint of surgeons is inefficiency. An inefficient OR not only frustrates them, but it wastes an enormous amount of money and leads to staff discontent. It often leads surgeons to start booking their cases elsewhere. An OR where the anesthesiologist looks at the chart and patient for the first time five minutes before a scheduled surgery can never hope to be efficient. A surgeon provided with different teams from day to day or even on the same day will never be efficient. An OR without an effective performance improvement team can never hope to improve.

Patient safety, successful surgery, and efficiency are critically important. The best way to achieve all three is to have standardized processes and a consistent OR and anesthesia team. Becoming efficient allows your surgeons to perform more cases per week and spend more time in their offices seeing prospective patients. This tantamount to adding additional orthopedic surgeons to your staff.

I am reminded of a hospital in Washington state that developed a destination joint center and incorporated its OR into the center. Its leaders created systems and teams and have reported cutting turnover times between total joints from 45 minutes to 11 minutes. The surgeon was bragging about it. It can be done.

Achieving Great Physician Relations

As noted in Jim Collins' well-known book *Good to Great,* greatness in business depends first on "getting the right people on the bus." This concept is just as critical in healthcare, especially in terms of getting the right physicians assembled for an orthopedic service line or destination center. There are four keys to determining the right physicians and getting them on your team:

- Specialization

- Strong physician relations

- Aligned goals

- Having a physician champion

Specialization

Naturally, subspecialty destination centers require surgeons who specialize. When I completed my orthopedic training in 1975, nearly every orthopedic surgeon was a generalist. Being a generalist meant that you could handle bone and joint surgery from the neck to the foot and everywhere in between. From trauma to back surgery, you were expected to be competent in every area. But generalization has become less popular with the advent of newer, more complex procedures and a host of new implants and techniques to go with them. Today, many orthopedic surgeons finishing residency spend another year in fellowship training in which they immerse themselves in one subspecialty area.

Patients look favorably upon subspecialization and even expect it. Often, when an individual needs care, he or she will go to great lengths to find the best spine surgeon, arthritis doctor, or knee expert. Although it is probably not necessary for all physicians to posses fellowship certificates, having surgeons focus their elective practice on a few areas is helpful when creating a subspecialty center. With the coming shortage of certain specialists, the development of a destination center is one of the best ways to recruit and showcase these specialty surgeons.

Strong Physician Relations

Without physicians to admit and care for patients, a hospital would sit empty and eventually disappear. But despite their critical role in hospital achievement, physicians are often taken for granted. By not showing an appreciation for physicians' skills, ideas, and concerns, you risk filling a hospital with physicians who are there physically but not emotionally. In contrast, physicians with the right attitude understand that collaboration with other physicians, as well as with the hospital, is the best way to improve care and create a superior reputation.

For hospitals to create healthy, collaborative doctor-management relationships, they must first understand the minds of physicians. When I visit a destination center and ask to see the latest physician satisfaction survey, I usually get blank looks. "We did one three years ago" is a common answer. In fairness, great physician relations are much more than satisfaction surveys or responding to complaints. I've been told that the first lesson in most hospital administration masters' programs is something along the lines of, "Don't anger the doctors." I've also been told it's the last point emphasized. Although I agree that angering the doctors is unlikely to foster strong relationships, acting simply out of fear isn't any more conducive to successful physician relations.

Historically, some physicians who sense this insecurity often use their power to intimidate administration, always threatening to leave if their demands aren't met. Feeling manipulated by the very professionals that they most need to collaborate with, administration may become passive-aggressive and even hostile. The physicians involved may characterize the administration as untrustworthy, uncaring, and incompetent—the so-called "dark side."

I've encountered many of these situations but find that most physicians don't leave the hospital because of them. Their practices are entrenched in the community and would be harmed by leaving, and the next hospital may not be any different. Within this cycle of mistrust, the tension escalates and becomes the predominate culture in the organization. Many administrators find themselves in this situation, put on the armor, and accept it as part of the job. It doesn't need to be that way.

Get to know people individually

Do you have a relationship with your physicians? Do you treat physicians as your most important customer? Does the amount of time you spend with individual physicians reflect this priority? How many have you met with one-on-one this year? How often do you meet with them? What do you talk about?

Many physicians will tell you that they have never spent any time with the leaders or other folks in the C-suite outside of being called in to discuss a problem. Seen primarily at large medical staff meetings, management becomes a "they" quite quickly. There is an obvious disconnect here. Despite being one of the hospital's most precious and perishable resources, the physicians get little or no individual attention. True relationships are individual, not in groups. If you are among those hospital administrators who connect with most of your physicians in a large group, you may not have optimal relationships.

Remember, even though CEOs see physicians weekly via the medical staff leadership structure, this is not the same as meeting with them individually. Often, the key physicians in your hospital, especially the entrepreneurial ones, do not get involved in medical staff leadership. They do not like the bureaucracy. They are out building surgical centers, MRI facilities, and physical therapy centers that often compete with you. All the medical staff leadership meetings in the world aren't going to help you develop working relationships with these very individuals who may be best suited to take your hospital and services to the next level.

Many administrators also assume that physicians would rather talk to one of their own, such as the chief medical officer (CMO). However, the CMO is not the boss—and physicians like to talk to the boss one-on-one. Spending time with the lead physician of a medical group does not translate to having a relationship with the other physicians in that group. Often, the docs in the group don't communicate well themselves. They may have their own issues of trust and often have different agendas. In fact, in orthopedics, a large percentage of new physician hires leave after two years.

So how can you create great relationships with your physicians? It depends on how serious you want to be. Consider meeting with your doctors one-on-one as an important first step. In this way, you can get to know them and understand how you can help them and how they can best help the organization. If hospital leaders spent 30 minutes three times per week meeting with doctors one-on-one, they could have 600 meetings per year. Put another way, leaders can substantially improve their relationships with physicians by committing just a small fraction of a typical 60-hour workweek.

Good leaders know that success depends not only on hospital-physician relations, but also on effective physician-physician relations. If the physicians are too competitive or adversarial, developing good hospital-physician relations will be that much more difficult. Any perceived favoritism toward one physician or another becomes a problem for administration. This is especially true in surgery, where physicians compete even more fiercely. Although the leader is not responsible for physician-physician relations, exploring ways to help is important.

Physicians who are distrustful of each other will work together in one of two situations. The first is when they have a common enemy. I would resist this approach, especially if you are the enemy. The more positive way to encourage collaboration is to create a common vision that benefits all. Creating a destination center can provide this common vision and help motivate physicians to work as a team.

Give and gain respect

Building a culture of respect must be a priority for any organization looking for superior service-line performance. It's important to understand the cultural differences between physicians and administrators. Administrators are generally group thinkers who spend a lot of time meeting and discussing. In a world where small margins and minor mistakes can have serious consequences, risk avoidance becomes very important. Administrators know their decisions usually become public, so often they will not make decisions quickly or at all. However, physicians may equate this approach with weakness or incompetence rather than due diligence. This is not helpful in creating good relations.

On the other hand, in clinical medicine, time is often of the essence. Physicians are action-oriented and must make decisions every day, even without all the facts. We are taught to listen to a problem, conduct a few tests, make a diagnosis, and start a treatment plan. This may occur within minutes of seeing the patient. Surgeons in the operating room often do this even more quickly. Administration may see physicians as impulsive.

Both cultures and views must be appreciated by both parties. They need each other. Leadership that recognizes these differences can address them directly. Gaining and giving respect goes a long way toward creating strong relations.

Transparency and trust

I have heard more than one story of administration telling physicians the hospital was losing money on a particular procedure, only to reveal later that the hospital did not possess accurate information, used creative accounting, or wasn't being completely truthful. This is a killer to healthy relationships with physicians. Withholding important information, particularly financial information that relates to physicians, is risky. Most physicians want to make the hospital money with their procedures. It gives them status within the hospital. And when given the full picture of hospital finances, top money-making docs will decrease their wasteful spending. Transparency engenders trust, and trust leads to better relations and a willingness to go the extra mile with you.

Align Your Goals

Phillip Ronning, in *Reinventing Centers of Excellence,* noted that physicians do not consider hospital success to be one of their top priorities. And hospital leaders, when asked about their highest priorities, rarely put physician success near the top. They often list capital projects, information technology, and other ventures. Clearly, physician and health system goals are not tightly aligned under most traditional models.

More hospitals today are attempting to align physician-hospital goals. Must-haves, such as a better patient experience, better patient outcomes, more volume, or a great reputation, are all goals around which you can begin to align and collaborate.

Financial goals are more difficult to align because hospitals and physicians are paid separately, giving physicians little incentive to try to reduce hospital costs, especially when doing so may mean changing vendors or lifelong clinical practices. However, a variety of models have been designed to help align physician and hospital goals, each with a unique set of pros and cons in the service-line arena:

- **Joint ventures** have been the most common arrangement between physicians and hospitals, usually related to an MRI machine or a surgical center. It is essentially a financial arrangement and does not necessarily align goals beyond the deal itself.

- **Gain sharing** allows physicians and hospitals to share any savings they realize. These savings must be achieved each year, so each year the bar is reset. The problem with this arrangement is that it's difficult to reduce costs enough in subsequent years to make a substantial difference.

- **Comanagement** agreements involve hospitals hiring a physician-owned company (usually composed of their own physicians) to manage the service line. Metrics are set regarding patient experience, outcomes, costs, and profitability. Compensation or continuation of the agreement usually depends on meeting the agreed-upon goals. Unfortunately, most hospitals lack the informational tools to help them create metrics and goals, and many physicians are not skilled in management. However, this arrangement has the potential to create the true alignment that is necessary for long-term success.

- **Hospital employment** of specialists is rapidly growing as an excellent way to align goals between doctors and management. I believe it will become

                                              Orthopedics and Spine

the most prevalent alignment method in the future. More and more, larger specialty groups, such as orthopedics and neurosurgery, are becoming employed. Younger surgeons are less likely to go out on their own today and are looking for employment. Older entrepreneurial surgeons who have built empires, including ancillaries, may be tiring of the constant rule changes and threats that abound daily. Hospitals that have developed good programs and good relationships with their physicians are in a perfect position to pursue this arrangement. Employment by itself, however, doesn't necessarily align all the goals or achieve the objectives. You must continue to take the steps noted previously to ensure the development of successful leadership and collaboration.

Create and Nurture Physician Champions

Hospitals cannot create a destination center for the physicians; they can only do it with them. Kyle Prickett, in his paper "Empowering and Mentoring Leadership: The Key to the Implementation of a New Delivery System for Care of Total Joint Patients,"[1] noted that a physician champion is the one ingredient that makes a program successful or unsuccessful. Champions are made, not born, although some are better suited for the role from the start.

Most physicians receive little or no leadership or business training during their medical education. Creating and mentoring physician champions can work wonders for your physician relations. Physician champions are usually energetic and highly skilled individuals. They command the respect of their peers. They may drive you crazy at times with their desire to do everything yesterday.

Helping your champions become leaders is important. Some hospitals have developed formal leadership programs with local universities, and others have paid for doctors to attend leadership conferences. There are other cost-effective ways to mentor. For example, create a book club with interested physicians, administration, and board members. Meet bimonthly or so to discuss various business and leadership books. Keep discussions about medical center issues off-limits, as there are plenty of other forums for that. Talk about concepts and ideas. The time you spend together as physicians, administrators, and board members discussing business and leadership issues and learning to relate to one another's worlds is more important than the books you read.

If you have the respect of these important physicians, they will carry the banner for you with the others. If you don't, your job will be that much tougher—if you are able to keep it.

Summary

Successful physician relationships and collaboration are critical to future success. Make the effort to get to know physicians individually, learn from them, teach them, create a vision with them, align your goals, be transparent, and gain and give respect. Relationship building is never easy, but it's essential.

Endnote

1. Kyle Prickett and Marshall K. Steele, MD. "Empowering and Mentoring Leadership: The Key to the Implementation of a New Delivery System for Care of Total Joint Patients," Marshall Steele & Associates, *www.marshallsteele.com/leadership.asp* (accessed April 15, 2009).

Understanding Vendor Relationships

Contributing writer: Judy Jones, MS

Physician-hospital alignment is pivotal, not only to development of service lines, but also to the transformation of healthcare. Another important but often untapped connection is the hospital-vendor relationship. The topic of vendor relationships is a tricky one. Vendors have products that affect patient, physician, and hospital performance. The success of these products for the patient, physician, and hospital ultimately determines the success of the vendor. Navigating these relationships is important. Are vendors friends or foes?

Most hospital administrators think of their vendors as cost centers rather than partners. Any conversation about orthopedic surgery is sure to include implant costs, which can consume 35%–60% of the reimbursement for a procedure. In rare cases, implant costs can wipe out the entire reimbursement. All costs, including implant costs, are integral to service-line profitability.

From the hospital's perspective and the literature, implants are often considered commodity items. Good results can be obtained from most of them. Therefore, it makes sense that prices should reflect this reality. When the hospital has tight margins or none at all, implant choice becomes topic No. 1 in reducing costs.

However, surgeons feel pressure from patients and even their peers to use the latest and greatest, even if proof of superiority is lacking. Each system is slightly different, creating a learning curve when change is made. Many physicians do not want to subject themselves and their patients to this learning curve unless real patient benefit can be realized.

The vendors all tout the unique benefits of their implants and their service. They stay until the case is over and work late into the night with the physician. In this way they earn the trust and loyalty of the physician.

The hospital that now wants a commodity price in spite of these realities can become a problem for the vendor and the physician. The hospital calls the vendor into the facility to discuss implant costs, claiming that joint replacement surgery has become unprofitable due to the cost of implants. The hospital's ultimatum to the vendor: Reduce prices or be excluded from our list of accepted companies.

The vendor representative is confused. The company had provided the hospital years of great service, state-of-the art technology, education, and 3 a.m. deliveries when necessary. The vendor wonders why he is being singled out as he observes so much waste every day in the operating room (OR). So the representative approaches the surgeon, with whom he's worked on hundreds of cases. The surgeon has not been given the information on reimbursement and costs. He may not be convinced that the hospital loses money on joint replacement. In fact, the vendor may produce information to the contrary. The surgeon sides with the vendor and tells the hospital administration that he will change hospitals if he cannot use these products.

Ill feelings occur between all parties involved. Trust is eroded. The hospital feels betrayed that the surgeon sided with the vendor when it has provided him with a great working environment. It also feels betrayed by the vendor, who is now interfering with the hospital-physician relationship. The surgeon thinks the hospital is not on his or the patients' side and is willing to reduce quality to save a few bucks. The classic catch-22 ensues: The hospital does not want to lose one of its top surgeons but does not feel it can continue on the present path; the surgeon doesn't want to leave the hospital but feels forced.

In case after case, one of three things happens:

1. The vendor reduces the product price (hospital wins, vendor loses). The vendor may then try work-arounds to the contract to avoid the effect of lower prices, which further angers the hospital and erodes trust.

2. The physician leaves (vendor wins short term, physician often loses, hospital loses).

3. The hospital gives in (hospital loses, vendor wins) and loses credibility for future negotiations. The vendor position is validated.

However, if you have great relationships with your vendors, scenarios in which one entity wins and another loses can be avoided.

Vendors' Role in Service Line Development

I was speaking at a conference recently at which a hospital's vice president (VP) relayed an interesting, more positive story. Although she had not run an OR prior to assuming the VP position several months earlier, it seemed obvious that the OR was not as efficient as it could be. So she sought outside experts to provide unbiased opinions.

What did she do? She looked to the hospital's top three orthopedic vendors for help. After all, these vendors had worked with the OR staff in dozens of hospitals around the state and would have seen all kinds of systems and protocols.

Her initial meeting with the vendors lasted more than four hours. The vendors' feedback not only reinforced her impression, but also provided valuable suggestions for improvement. Following such immediate success, the hospital continues to hold frequent meetings with the vendors on a variety of topics to share information, solicit feedback, and seek continued improvements. Vendors can be important partners not only to surgeons, but to hospitals as well.

Hospital support

Some vendors have bought, created, or partnered with companies that provide services to hospitals to help them become more effective and efficient in caring for the patients. These services are usually focused on the hospital care of patients who are receiving implants for joints, spine, fractures, sports, foot/ankle, and hand. These services are separate fee-for-service arrangements outside of the fees for the implants. Hospitals that are more effective and cost-efficient are better for our healthcare system and better for the vendors as well. By leading this effort, vendors show their commitment to healthcare. However, their motives in doing so are often questioned by hospitals that have not had excellent vendor relationships and view the effort as self-serving.

Physician involvement

One item on which hospitals, physicians, and vendors all agree is that the reimbursement for procedures involving significant implant use should be higher. The development of implants in orthopedic surgery and spine has created incredible value for the public. However, in the past several years, implant costs have risen faster than hospital and surgeon reimbursement. Vendors' margins have consistently exceeded those of hospitals. This has created stress between vendors and hospitals as hospital margins shrink. Efforts to improve third-party payments have been less than successful. Medicare, the major payer for total joints, doesn't negotiate, and other private payers typically follow the government payer's lead.

Physicians are at the center of this issue. The normal economics of capitalism don't work in this relationship. In capitalism, the purchaser and the user are usually the same, giving the purchaser leverage to walk away if the price cannot be agreed on. In hospital economics, physicians order the product and the hospital pays. Because of the medical culture's emphasis on quality, the last thing any physician wants to do is compromise care to achieve cost savings. Many surgeons are uncomfortable negotiating prices.

Complicating all this is the fact that most physicians do not personally measure and aggregate the results of their surgeries. The literature on surgery success is usually contributed by experts, many of whom are implant developers or have relationships with that industry. Complications of the procedure are measured by the hospital, but these don't clearly correlate to implant selection. Because of the myriad variables involved—surgeon skill, patient health, and so on—it is extremely difficult to determine whether implant selection affects results.

For example, if you ask Tiger Woods to hit your driver and the ball goes 300 yards, you really can't say those are your results. If he hits everyone's driver 300 yards, then the drivers are equal in this regard. Understanding the complexities of the work, physicians are often reluctant to question their peers' judgment, particularly relating to implants. In the same way, they do not want others questioning theirs.

Hospitals' true implant costs, reimbursement, and profitability are not customarily shared with physicians. So when a hospital tells the surgeon that it is losing money, the surgeon may discount this assertion. To have a good partner, you need to be a good partner. Transparency goes a long way in making this happen.

Don't merely call a meeting on implant costs

One aspect of being a good partner is to ask how you can help before you begin asking for help. Unless you've addressed the physicians' concerns, don't call a meeting on implant costs. You will be given a list of their needs and issues longer than yours. When their vendor shows up at 2 a.m. for a case and you haven't addressed long-standing physician concerns, you are at a huge disadvantage. You must create a system and partnership in which physicians' issues are continuously discussed and solved. This creates trust and an awareness that you care about their issues as well. Only then should you broach your concerns, including the subject of implant costs.

You must also understand that surgeons become comfortable with products and dislike change and the adaptation time that goes along with developing skill with a new one. Realize that the surgeon is loyal not only to the vendor, but to the product as well. Think of it this way: You've been using Windows-based computers for years. The company decides to switch to Apple-based computers because they are cheaper. Everything is different. During that learning curve, everything takes longer to do. It is uncomfortable, inefficient, and unfamiliar. You even make a few mistakes and lose some data. Surgeons do not like to involve their patients in a learning curve if it can be avoided.

Value and quality

Hospitals need healthy contribution margins to grow and meet the expanding needs of patients. For most of my career, quality trumped everything. Cost was just not part of the conversation. The concept of value—quality divided by cost—was never really discussed. But value must become a part of our medical culture if we are to succeed. For example, if implants are a commodity with comparable results, the lowest price provides the best value. However, if an implant can be proven to last twice as long, making the chance for revision 90% lower, it is more valuable and should command a higher price. But unless the payer recognizes this value, the hospital and the vendor have a problem.

Unfortunately, when vendors offer newer products with the promise of superior performance, usually little clinical data exist that show superiority, and payers subsequently refuse to pay more. If we hope to succeed long term, we must help physicians understand the concept of value and why this does not undermine quality in any way. We must also help payers understand that higher quality can be cost-effective and provide more value.

Role of the vendor

Orthopedic device vendors do more than merely sell their products. Consider their list of responsibilities:

- Train surgeons on the use of their products

- Introduce hospitals, surgeons, and the public to new technology

- Help surgeons plan individual cases, including implant selection

- Train OR staff members on use of products being used for individual procedures

- Provide education for patients on the products and the surgical procedures through product brochures and hospital Web sites

- Deliver the equipment on time, every time

In addition to these tasks, surgeons rely on vendors to provide knowledge and support within and outside the OR. Remember, the vendor representative has seen many different cases, and surgeons deal with unusual or difficult situations. He or she can share how other surgeons handled similar cases or give the name of the surgeon with whom to consult. If necessary, vendors can call their corporate office or the designer surgeons for additional support. All this support is critical to comfort and confidence of the surgeon as well as the result for the patient.

Surgical scheduling

Once a case is scheduled at the hospital, the OR staff communicates with the vendor to be sure that the equipment is ordered for the case. For busy surgeons performing multiple procedures in one day, it is essential that there are enough sets of hospital instrumentation. Also, it is critical to schedule same-type cases throughout the day so the instruments can be sent to central sterile and returned for the next case. This takes coordination among the surgeon's office, the hospital scheduling staff, and the vendor.

Staff training

Vendors often provide training on the newest technology for the OR staff and the floor staff, which enhances case efficiency. These learning sessions discuss the technology, instrumentation, research results, and techniques. The floor staff learns how the new technology may assist in recovery, as well as any precautions that should be followed with the new product.

Equipment management and delivery

The vendor is also responsible for the delivery of the necessary equipment and the implants prior to the day of the procedure. For the most part, orthopedic cases are elective procedures, so the surgeon and the representative plan the case in advance. They must ensure that the equipment is delivered and logged into the system during the time frame required by the hospital to sterilize and prepare the equipment for the case. Any delay in delivery will delay the surgery, leading to increased costs in addition to surgeon, employee, and patient dissatisfaction. No vendor wants to be responsible for dissatisfaction.

Emergency cases

As noted, most cases are planned in advance. However, there are sometimes changes in the schedule and/or type of equipment needed, especially for emergency cases such as trauma and fractures. The vendor must respond to the surgeon's need, sometimes in the wee hours. Surgeries cannot be accomplished without the necessary equipment. Therefore, for the surgeon, the representative is a trusted colleague who can be depended on at all times. He or she is also a valued member of the hospital's OR team.

New technology

Vendors call surgeons into their offices frequently to update knowledge and to introduce new equipment. Every surgeon wants to be updated on industry standards and new products that will provide better outcomes for his or her patients. The vendor also provides best-practice knowledge, studies, and articles.

This relationship may differ greatly from the interaction that surgeons have with administrators. Far too many surgeons have commented that the hospital CEO has never made a visit to his or her office.

Surgeon training

Surgeons receive continuous training to perform procedures such as joint replacement, fracture repair, spine and sports procedures, and so on. To receive training, surgeons travel with their vendor representative—the expert on the utilization of the equipment—to corporate headquarters or regional training courses to learn best-practice techniques. During this experience and throughout each procedure, the physician and vendor rely on each other to succeed, creating an understandably strong bond.

For surgeons to be proficient, they must have multiple opportunities to gain continuing medical education credits and become versed in the latest technology. All vendors provide educational programs designed for healthcare professionals. The aim is to improve their knowledge, enhance their understanding of innovative surgical techniques, and present the latest in biomedical research and development.

Patient education

Many implant companies offer educational tools designed to help patients understand the surgery better. Also, because efficiency is a key issue in every orthopedic office, these patient education materials help streamline patients' office experiences by engaging them in education during waiting periods and exam times. Patients are encouraged to read brochures, watch videos, and browse wall hangings that answer many common questions about particular ailments and their treatment. Educated patients tend to have a better understanding of their conditions and their role in healing.

Patient education materials provided by vendors may include the following:

- Posters

- Drawings/photos of pre- and postoperative hips, knees, and shoulders

- Brochures addressing FAQs

- Models of the joints with the implants

- Videos explaining procedures

By using these materials, the surgeon ensures that every patient receives a complete and consistent explanation of his or her condition and its treatment options. The surgeon also saves time and energy by not having to repeat the same information all day, every day.

Some vendors also offer marketing support to surgeons' practices in the form of:

- Web site design and updates

- PowerPoint presentations

- Seminar templates for public forums

Negotiating price

Most vendors believe that their product is superior to the competition's, but they all can't be right. Although hospitals recognize that there are differences in the various products, they believe that similar products should be priced accordingly. In a commodity situation, price and service are the only variables. Determining whether you have a commodity situation can be very controversial. Strategies that hospitals can use to obtain the best value when purchasing implants are discussed next.

Value-based pricing

Create a value committee cochaired by the medical director of the subspecialty and director of materials management. These cochairs should then select other members. The committee should meet quarterly or as necessary to discuss surgeon preference items such as implants, new requests, and other concerns. Surgeons and/or vendors should be invited to the meeting to make their case to the committee based on the evidence or other important factors.

The value committee should consider the following:

- Place each implant type into use-dependent categories:

  - Standard primary implants (use in most patients)

  - Nonstandard primary implants (use in selected patients with unusual requirements)

  - Special implants (unis, patellofemoral, etc.)

- Use published outcome data on specific implants to determine whether differences exist

- Evaluate all current vendor implant costs and compare them with one another and against national benchmark data when available

- Determine whether price variation is justified for a specific implant in the same category

- Set the price for each implant

- Determine implant volume for each type and vendor

The cochairs should then discuss these recommendations with the surgeons and get their input.

The advantages to this approach are:

- Surgeons participate in the discussion

- Vendors have a chance to participate in the discussion

- Decisions are more evidence-based

- Preference may be maintained

- Surgeon acceptance is more likely

The disadvantages are:

- Skillful negotiation is required

- Vendors may not agree to pricing

- Surgeons may not be willing to support pricing and/or change of implants

- Staff members must learn about and store multiple vendor products

- Some consensus on demand matching may be required

For example, an 85-year-old woman may not need the same implant as a 50-year-old athletic man. If the surgeon does not agree, this type of program will fail, as all the implants will be in the higher price category.

Capped pricing

In this scenario, implants are considered equal without going through the rigors of evidence. Value is determined in a less scientific manner, with the focus on costs. The committee structure is the same. Its responsibilities include:

- Determining national benchmarks for pricing of certain implants

- Setting one price for all like implants (e.g., variable axis screws, primary hips)

The advantages of this approach are:

- Less complicated than the parameters of the value committee

- Flexibility for surgeon to use any vendor

The disadvantages are:

- Vendors may not agree to pricing

- Vendors may leverage surgeons

- Surgeons may not agree

- More vendors may be involved

- OR staff members will need to be trained to learn the utilization of multiple systems as well as provide storage for more equipment

Restricted vendor policy

In this situation, the hospital asks for a request for proposal from a variety of vendors. The number of vendors will be restricted, thus increasing their potential volume. The concept is that with higher volume, the price should be lower, as total profit to the vendor should not change. Although it sounds simple, this approach is one of the most difficult to implement.

The advantages to this approach are:

- Reduced vendors will improve OR efficiency

- Costs can be kept down

The disadvantages are:

- Surgeons may be upset by the need to change vendors

- Hospital-surgeon relations may suffer

- Surgeons may become uncooperative or leave

Summary

Not all hospitals will benefit from the coming barrage of musculoskeletal care needs over the next 10 years. Vendor relationships, like surgeon relationships, need not be acrimonious. Vendors can be a great source of information and support. They can help you create happier, healthier patients; a better reputation; and a more profitable service line. If your vendors and surgeons do not share these ideals, you are at a huge disadvantage.

Addressing the concerns of the patients and physicians in a consistent, reliable way will get you on your way to gaining physician support. Being transparent with physicians is critical to developing trust. Considering all costs and waste will give you credibility. A hospital that does all this and has a relationship of mutual respect and interest with its vendors and physicians has a better chance to capitalize on the future demand than one that does not.

This is a tricky topic. It takes two committed parties to create a relationship, but it will not succeed every time. Some folks on both sides are very short-term oriented and will constantly try for win-lose outcomes. Both parties will decide whether vendors are friends or foes. There are some competing interests. If you do succeed in becoming friends and strive toward mutual benefit, you will be ahead of the game, and your patients will be rewarded as well.

Secrets to Extraordinary Marketing

Contributing writers: Anthony Cirillo, FACHE, ABC, Andrea Mastry, BA

"Build it and they will come," the saying goes. But if you don't build what they want, no one will come. If you don't tell them about how it meets their needs, only some will come. If you don't meet their needs better than your competitor, very few will come. If you don't communicate to the right people at the right time in the right way, you won't find success. If you can do all these things, you will establish a viable destination center of superior performance.

Marketing Doesn't Equal Advertising

Many healthcare professionals believe marketing means advertising. They run huge advertising campaigns about their centers, "paint the shack" as self-proclaimed centers of excellence, and make claims that are met perhaps 10% of the time.

There are several problems with claims advertising:

- You may inadvertently set an expectation that is difficult to meet. The very best form of marketing comes from word-of-mouth referrals from satisfied patients. One of the keys to obtaining word of mouth is exceeding expectations.

- This type of advertising diverts important resources away from under-standing customers' needs and improving your services.

- If you rely on advertising, you must keep doing it—and that's expensive.

- This form of advertising is unfocused and provides no intrinsic value. In fact, I once saw two hospitals advertising on opposite sides of the same bus, both making similar claims. They got you coming and going, so to speak.

You must make people aware of what you are doing, but advertising is just one of many aspects of marketing.

The Marketing Mindset

When I speak at meetings, I often ask, "Who here is from marketing?" Inevitably, only a few hands out of 100 or so go up. These people think of marketing as a department. The correct response would have been for every hand to be raised. Everyone in the hospital is a marketer. Creating the right mindset is important. Here are a few ideas.

 Orthopedics and Spine

Make marketing everyone's job

Because marketing is about discovering and fulfilling needs and communicating abilities, it belongs to everyone. Staff members and even volunteers can serve as integral marketing resources. Keeping them up to date on the progress of the program will empower them to discuss and market your programs.

Provide talking points. Use the employee newsletter to update staff when major milestones are accomplished, such as naming your spine care coordinator or physician leader, updates on renovations, and announcing the opening date of the center. Internal newsletters do not need to be monthly, but certainly frequent enough to keep the positive buzz in the air. Memos from the CEO and paycheck stuffers are other good ways to keep employees informed.

Don't forget vendors and product suppliers who are in the hospital every day. They are often trusted by the public to tell them where to go. These people need to be aware of your services so they can be spokespeople for the hospital as well.

Walk in your customers' shoes

Understand what customers want, rather than what you want; understand their concerns, not just yours. For example, in recruiting a spine surgeon, you may discover a concern you never considered, such as career opportunities for the surgeon's spouse. When you know the concern, you can address it. Understand that people need you at different times. The patient with severe arthritis of the knee or hip needs you now. However, the baby boomer with some discomfort might not need you for a long time. Do you market only for the immediate return on investment, or do you market for the longer-term return?

As an orthopedic surgeon, I was often referred patients with arthritis who didn't need surgery at the time. Many surgeons tell such patients not to return until they need surgery. However, I learned that providing excellent nonoperative care to patients was one of the key components to developing a successful surgical practice. Developing many nonoperative options for these patients and keeping track of them allowed me to stay in contact and provide any new advice or treatments that surfaced. With an emphasis on consumer needs, you create trust. Trust creates loyalty, loyalty creates a lifetime of business.

Understand that different markets mean different needs. Who is the target audience of McDonald's? Look around. They have Happy Meals with toys. Their market is kids, and they are fully aware of that. Another way of looking at this is thinking in terms of market segments. You would not advertise in *The New York Times* if your market area is Peoria. I wouldn't send a direct-mail piece for total joints to someone under 50 who is not likely to need this service.

However, sending a sports medicine piece makes sense, especially given the fact that most sports medicine patients are in their 40s and 50s. I always said I stood on the sidelines at high school football games not necessarily to take care of the student athletes, but to take care of their parents in the stands.

Create Your Brand

What is the difference between marketing and branding? Marketing is something you do: Find out what the needs are, help create a better product, and communicate its value. Branding is something that is done to you by the public. Try as you might, you cannot really brand yourself. You certainly can decide how you would like to be branded and create the programs to support this, but ultimately you are branded by others. What they think and what they say becomes your brand. It is the culmination of your efforts to understand patient needs, create better systems of care, and communicate your unique selling proposition (USP). If you don't have a brand, the creation of destination centers is a powerful way to begin one.

Most of the marketing and educational materials you develop will require a name, logo, and theme. Therefore, you will need to create these early when establishing a destination center. Think regionally. The South Florida Regional Joint Replacement Center might be better than a more local name. Either use the hospital logo or create a unique logo for the center. The theme can also be tied to all your marketing and patient education materials.

One hospital created a group room that looked like a tropical island. The wall-paper had white sandy beaches, deep blue water, and swaying palm trees. A few lounge chairs lined the room for family members and patients to sit on, and during group lunch they were served chicken with mango salsa, and the drinks had little umbrellas in the cups. A piece of driftwood with "Cabana Room" written on it was hung outside the group room.

Other theme examples include sports, luxury spa, outdoor adventure, and a hotel-like atmosphere. With a unique name, logo, and theme, you have a better chance to be remembered and create a brand.

The Marketing Plan

A marketing plan combines all the issues previously mentioned. That plan must be tied to organizational goals, based on sound and current data, and developed not only by the marketing department but in conjunction with other key service personnel. It must have achievable goals and measurable results, with assigned, time-sensitive responsibilities. Keep in mind that a plan cannot be successful without budgeting is a research component so that you start to understand the underlying needs of your key audiences. Remember that your customers include not only patients, but also referring physicians, specialists, and payers. Think about marketing to their needs as well.

One of the obvious issues is identifying who your customers are. In this section we will discuss the referring physician/specialist, the patient, and the payers.

Referring physicians

Relationships and communication remain the essential tools for engaging referring physicians. Information collection and relationship building is more than an item on a to-do list; it is about creating a culture in the organization of understanding what your customers want and how to deliver it. When you understand what motivates them, you can begin to influence their decisions. This information can then be leveraged to influence others as well. It's about building relationships and providing value.

The primary care physician (PCP) is usually the first person a patient sees about a problem. Patients trust their PCPs and seek their advice. Just as consumers choose their PCPs through word of mouth, PCPs rely on word of mouth to choose their specialists. Word of mouth drives referrals most of the time. What should your strategy be for primary care? How do we get PCPs to send their musculoskeletal patients to our specialists? Organizations that collect data on prospects can understand the experiences and needs of their customers and directly target their marketing efforts.

Other valuable marketing resources in the community are the various primary care and orthopedic specialists' offices. For years, pharmaceutical companies have understood that direct-to-consumer marketing in physicians' offices has a tremendous payoff. However, hospitals traditionally have not taken advantage of the access to potential customers that the physicians' waiting room presents. Begin branding the new program by building relationships with physician offices and using their office space to display program-specific materials.

Primary care physicians

Your care coordinator can act as a spokesperson and meet with PCPs and orthopedic specialists or their practice managers to talk about your center before the program launch date and on an ongoing basis thereafter. Physician visits provide an opportunity to ask for program feedback and to build stronger relationships.

The following are a few ideas to connect with referring physicians and their staff:

- **Find out who they are.** Make sure your organization asks patients not only who their surgeon is but who their PCP is when registering. Create a strategic grid that lists all of the PCPs and their history with you and your specialists. Estimate their total referral potential and how much your specialists are capturing. How do their referrals stack up with their colleagues?

- **Make their priority your priority.** The more you know about your referrer, the more you can discern their priorities and create relationships with them. You need to develop not only a professional relationship with patients but a personal one as well. The same is true among physicians and between administrators and physicians. Be friendly with as many people as possible. Ask them about themselves. People like to do business with their friends.

- **Hire a physician liaison.** A physician liaison can find out what you are doing right and what you are doing wrong. Have him or her visit the primary care offices and develop a relationship with the office staff and the office manager. Find out what they need. The liaison should meet with the physician if possible. If not, make a list of questions the office staff can ask him or her. Create profiles of the offices you visited and review them each week with the leadership of the service lines.

- **Give something away that is professionally valuable.** Within reason and within the law, there is nothing like giving something valuable away that will help colleagues care for their patients. PCPs appreciate having educational tools for their patients. Providing them tools such as a "Top 10 Things to Do for Arthritis/Back Pain" pamphlet is very helpful. Write the dates, times, and locations of your educational seminars on a business card or brochure they can give to their patients. After you have created your nonoperative physical therapy programs for patients, you should inform your PCPs of the content and locations, complete with a referral pad.

- **Facilitate meetings between specialists and PCPs.** In today's world of hospitalists, specialists rarely interact personally with PCPs. Traditional brown bag lunch and learns for physicians and their office staff are powerful.

- **Create an "easy pass system" for patients.** With an easy pass, access and waiting is improved. Many organizations make referrals unnecessarily difficult. When I was practicing, I ordered many MRIs. To try to make getting an appointment easy for my patients, I asked my secretary to schedule the appointment while the patient was in the office. If she got a recording at the first office she called, she'd move on to a competitor who would answer the phone and schedule an appointment.

- **Use technology to communicate.** The 2009 stimulus package has real incentives for physicians to adopt new technology. Aid physicians by helping them conceive and launch their electronic medical record system. Further, automate referrals online and establish a secure physician portal with a platform to complain, make suggestions, and so on. Finally, automate your system to help you provide prompt reports. But don't forget to pick up the telephone.

Specialists

Understanding and meeting the needs of your PCPs is critical for getting patients referred to your specialists. However, it is your specialists that bring most of the patients to your hospital for surgery, interventions, and ancillaries. If you don't understand and meet the needs of your specialists, your PCP strategy will not be fruitful.

Knowing your referring specialists is much easier than knowing your primary physicians; however, the approach should be similar. In addition to the strategies noted previously, you must do the following:

- Capture data:

    - Number of procedures performed

    - Number of patients admitted

    - Types of procedures

    - Total revenue produced

    - Payer types

    - ZIP codes

    - Primary care names matched to surgeons

    - Estimate of total potential

- Provide an efficient operating/interventional room. The No. 1 complaint of surgeons and interventionalists is lack of efficiency. If you fail to create a safe and efficient operating room, you risk losing your physicians.

- Provide their patients with an extraordinary hospital experience. Physicians are tired of apologizing to patients for poor experiences they have in hospitals. This was the main reason that I developed the destination center concept. Creating a destination center will not only create loyal physicians,

                                                      Orthopedics and Spine

but it will make recruitment much easier. Where would a specialist rather work: a destination center or a traditional hospital setting? The answer is easy.

- Start capturing the results of their interventions. Most physicians do not measure and aggregate the results of their surgeries and interventions. One way you can help them while helping yourself is to begin capturing this information on all elective patients who have had interventions or surgery, as described in Chapter 2.

- Provide patient amenities. To generate buzz regarding your center, decide which amenities you would like to offer patients. For example, some programs send each patient a rose with a signed card from the surgeon and the staff at the center. Others bring a warmed, wet towel each afternoon to the patient, creating a first-class atmosphere. Offer a gourmet meal the night before the patient and his or her coach (a family member charged with aiding in recovery, as described in Chapter 4) leave the hospital. T-shirts or tote bags are common gifts. The possibilities are endless.

- Ask for physician feedback. Many hospitals conduct periodic physician surveys of the entire staff, but these may not be focused enough to help you identify the real issues. Meet with specialists regularly one-on-one to get the real scoop. Do it before they ask for a meeting with you to complain.

Patients

Most marketing efforts and money go toward the patients. When you are developing a musculoskeletal center, you will inevitably be caring for patients of all ages.

For total joint patients, the average age is 70. In sports, hands, foot/ankle, joints, or spine, the average age is in the mid-50s. The oldest baby boomers are now 62, and most of your marketing efforts will be directed toward them (see "The Consumer the Boomer," later in this chapter).

If you become a destination center like the top players—the Mayo and Cleveland Clinics of the world—there is every possibility that people will call you directly and self-refer. Are you ready? Set up systems to accommodate self-referral. If you have a call center, set up protocols. If not, be transparent, profile your physicians on the hospital's Web pages, and include an e-mail contact. Also, consider setting up an informational Webinar for interested patients.

Payers

Payers are customers. Payers are not merely insurance companies, but also the employers that are footing the bill. If you are creating a hand or spine center, a relationship with workers' compensation carriers is also important because they will direct patients. Hand and back injuries are a huge issue for them.

Many hospitals, after developing an inpatient destination center, discover their costs fall and their patients are going home rather than to skilled nursing facilities. This is a tremendous savings for insurance companies. However, insurance companies are always reluctant to direct patients on cost alone. How can you leverage this to your advantage? The best way is to ask your patients at various time intervals after their surgery whether the surgery was successful. Once you demonstrate quality, insurance companies will be more likely to direct patients your way if you are also the most cost-effective option.

Competitor Analysis

A plan cannot be written in a vacuum. You need to understand who your competitors are, including their strengths and weaknesses. That is not as easy as it sounds. If you view yourself solely as a local hospital, your competitors are pretty clearly defined. But if you are creating a destination center, you need to consider your competitors on a broader scale. The hospital you are competing with may be in an adjoining county, state, or region, or in another part of the country.

What is the competition doing better?

Competition is good because it makes you strive to be better. You need to know and learn from your competition. Find out what your competitors are doing and what the best organizations are doing. If they are better, you need to understand why. Sometimes all you need to do is ask. Proud employees will readily share this information with you. The next best way is to ask the patients who go there. Patients often came back to me for minor problems after having a major procedure at my competitor. Simply asking why they went there and what they experienced is a great way to find out what the competition is doing better.

For example, some patients told me they went elsewhere because they thought they would get a better result. However, I quickly learned that the surgeons at those hospitals had not provided information on the results. This perception of better results was not necessarily a reality. I had no results to show them either and could only position myself as an excellent surgeon—not prove it. It was then that I decided to collect my results and share them with patients. This demonstrated to my patients that results were important to me and gave me an advantage over competitors who did not have results to share.

Be willing to hear the truth

Most marketing departments don't feel that they have permission to tell the clinical professionals that the competition is better. Criticizing them and the current hospital service might sound like disloyalty and cause them to be defensive and angry. Professionals might think that it is marketing's job to tell the public we are better, not to tell us that we are not.

This needs to change. Marketing needs to find out what others are doing and should be encouraged to tell the truth. Only by facing the stark reality of each situation can you hope to do better.

Identify your unique selling proposition

Patients will choose you over the competition if they are drawn to your USP. By all means, strive to have more than one. Telling consumers that you have great nurses or doctors is not a USP. That is the message of every hospital I've been to, and there is nothing unique about it. When we started our center at Anne Arundel Medical Center, we focused on the uniqueness of the experience. We did such a good job that one day, about three months after opening, a patient remarked that this was not like a hospital experience, but more like being at camp. Thus, the name "Joint Camp" was coined, not by a smart marketing person but by a patient. This became our USP.

We later decided that this wasn't enough and began measuring the results of our interventions a year after surgery. Now we had two unique selling propositions—experience and outcomes. To be successful in creating a destination center, you need to have a USP that your patients value.

Transparency

There is a growing movement toward transparency in all things healthcare—quality and pricing being the two obvious levelers. But most consumers do not know how to interpret or use quality indicators, so spending tens of thousands of dollars on the right to use some rating company's data is probably not a strategy worth pursuing. That does not mean third-party endorsements are bad. For example, The Joint Commission has a certification program in musculoskeletal programs.

Quality means different things to different people. Quality to the consumer might be the sum of the experience, whereas quality to the PCP is a specific metric. Know what is important to each audience. With more patients lacking insurance, carrying greater self-pay burdens, and considering medical tourism, price becomes a major factor in decisions. Hospitals such as Geisinger Medical Center in Pennsylvania guarantee their heart surgeries, just like a car warranty. Are you prepared to guarantee your work?

Communicating with the Right Medium

A Harris Interactive survey of 4,220 baby boomers found outright annoyance with television advertising. Only 3% are extremely satisfied with television advertising, and 66% believe ads have gotten crude and are unlikely to purchase something if they find the advertising offensive. According to the ad agency Millennium, 60% of those over age 50 believe that advertising aimed at them presents them as infirm or immobile; 75% of those over 50 think the only products specifically targeted at them are life insurance products, false teeth, and incontinence or sexual fixes. Two-thirds believe ads are targeted to those under 40. Yet 36% of hospital marketing budgets are devoted to advertising, with just 4% of that devoted to online efforts.

The Web

One of the first entry points into the hospital is the Web site. Your destination center should be prominent. Consider the following:

- Create a positive impression at the first click. Your images and your words paint a picture of the experience. For example, type *www.celilo.org* into your browser. Look at the images. Not typical for a hospital's cancer site. This little 60-bed hospital attracts cancer patients from a seven-state area.

- Make it user-friendly. Make sure the font is large enough to read and that the elements are organized thoughtfully. Avoid forcing visitors to download a file to read it.

- Tape audio and video patient testimonials and place them prominently on your site and on YouTube and other sharing sites (with permission).

- Hire a search engine optimization company to position your center at the top of the search engine results for people seeking joint replacements. Google these terms yourself and see what comes up.

- Gather information about visitors to your site. Consider putting a bone and joint quiz or questionnaire for people to fill out. Initially collect the visitors' names and e-mail addresses and ask permission to send them further information.

- Post a patient blog that documents that person's experience.

- Produce a video that documents the experience from prehospital to postoperative. Lancaster (PA) General provides a virtual tour to patients as an example.

- If you have patient events, film a reunion, a luncheon, or a dinner. This shows the social benefits to participating in your program: friendships and fun.

- Foster community. Get permission to post joint patients' names in a password-protected area so they can communicate with one another after the hospital stay. To complement this, start a community forum where patients can post questions and others can answer.

Television

Television can be effective. Marketing consultant Kurt Medina suggests you start with a three- to four-second message that's not important, because viewers will likely miss it anyway. Use voiceover and graphics to support the message. Keep repeating one or two simple points. And be respectful. A hospital in Indiana uses television to educate and communicate with the public. Once a year, employees set up a forum in three segments:

- Do I need the surgery?

- What can I expect with the surgery?

- What can I expect after surgery?

They take live call-ins from the community and answer questions on-air.

Brochures

A service line brochure will help market the hospital's orthopedic and spine servic-es. The brochure can be distributed at seminars and other speaking engagements. This collateral piece can also be displayed at surgeons' offices, PCP offices, senior centers, extended care facilities, home health agencies, and in the hospital lobby. A service line brochure should be produced and ready to use before the launch of the program.

Community education and seminars

Many hospitals have community education events such as balance screenings, which focus on minimizing slips and falls and therefore broken hips and bones. Osteoporosis screenings and walking clubs also promote healthy bones and joints and can tie in with your orthopedic service line.

Seminars offered by the hospital and presented by a clinical professional can be a great way to engage the community. Physicians, care coordinators, and other speakers may take turns speaking throughout the year. The seminars are intended to educate the community while showcasing the service line. Surgeon appointments for interested attendees can be made at the close of the seminar if the partnering physicians are willing to reserve open appointment times for seminar attendees. Twenty percent of attendees typically book appointments with a specialist at the end of the seminar. Fifty percent of those who see a specialist typically end up choosing to have surgery. Hospitals can expect that, on average, 10% of the seminar attendees will eventually schedule surgery.

Seminars should be held a minimum of once per month. Consider holding seminars more often if attendance is larger than 20–25 people, as attendees within smaller groups are more likely to book surgery. Seminars should be held routinely at the hospital campus. This eliminates the need to rent a conference room or hall and presents the opportunity to cross-sell other hospital services and specialties. Additional seminars can be held off-site in surrounding communities. Orthopedic specialists' satellite offices are favorable seminar locations and may be used on days when patients are not being seen.

Food or other substantial refreshments do not need to be served at the seminar. Experience shows that providing meals often attracts community members with a different agenda. Attendees who are serious about getting help for their pain will come to a seminar even when no food is provided.

Community open house

Holding an open house for the community and media is a grand way to generate awareness for the new center. This event should be held several weeks after the launch date, once the initial program opportunities have been worked out and after several patients have experienced the new center. Patient testimonials to the media will be extremely powerful.

The care coordinator and the surgeons can ask staff members to identify patients who have an interesting story to tell. Arrange for these patients to attend your open house and speak with the media whenever possible.

Word-of-Mouth Strategies

Word of mouth is the best and most enduring strategy you can employ. In effect, word of mouth defines your brand. Hugely successful brands such as Starbucks and Harley Davidson seldom advertise. Why? Because they understand and leverage word of mouth by following these principles:

- **Create extraordinary experiences.** With free Internet access in its cafés, Starbucks has created an experience, not just coffee. We must create these experiences in healthcare. When you consider the whole package, the end experience, and bundle accordingly, you create an emotional attachment with customers. If any part of a hospital stay goes awry, it affects the overall experience. That is why forward-thinking hospitals, such as Cleveland Clinic, have hired the new CEO—a chief experience officer (a physician)—to look at the whole patient experience.

- **Create community.** Shouldice Hospital in Canada has an annual reunion dinner for patients. The hospital's word of mouth accounts for 96% of admissions. Many joint and spine centers hold monthly patient reunion lunches. These are hosted by the surgeons and nurses. They provide the opportunity for patients to reunite with their caregivers and each other in a social situation. Other centers host annual events as well.

- **Bring physicians together.** In medicine, just like in any other industry, people do business with people who they know and trust. Create opportunities for your medical staff to get together. Grand rounds, happy hours, golf outings, and family gatherings provide the opportunity for doctors to get to know one another and learn about the expertise within the hospital community.

- **Adopt an important cause.** Adopt a cause, such as fall prevention, osteoporosis education, or exercise for seniors, and bring in the specialists and PCPs as partners. Keeping patients healthy and out of your hospital promotes trust. When someone really needs your services, who do you think they will choose? The specialist who was trying to sell his services or the one who was trying to help?

- **Create partners.** Make the community your partner as well. The high school coaches association is a great way to begin building trust with local coaches. Give them seminars, materials, and books. Stand on the sidelines yourself. Don't stop there. Giving a talk at the beginning of each sports season on the prevention and treatment of injuries is a valued service. We provided every youth coach a copy of my book *Sideline Help* as part of their education. These are inexpensive ways to provide value back to the community and begin creating your brand. Health clubs are always looking for speakers as well. Teaching golfers how to avoid back problems or skiers how best to avoid knee injuries is another way to build goodwill and demonstrate your expertise. Don't forget the Arthritis Foundation. If you don't have a chapter in your community, start one. One hospital I visited donated an office just off the main reception area to the Arthritis Foundation. Patients coming to the office for educational materials from the Arthritis Foundation went into the front lobby of the hospital. That's what I call brilliant.

- **Monitor the environment.** People are talking about you. Do you know who they are, how to respond, and how to leverage what they are saying? Establish Google Alerts for keywords such as your orthopedic practice name, hospital name, physician names, and others. Track the results. You may uncover a physician ambassador or, conversely, someone who was displeased with you. Engage them and respond. Of course this has consumer implications as well. To participate in the discussion, start a physician blog and publicize it to referrers. Blogs humanize the experience.

The Consumer the Boomer

There is one patient segment that deserves special attention: the baby boomer. This demographic will dominate healthcare for the next 30 years. There are 78 million baby boomers, and one in six will have significant arthritis. Every third boomer will be overweight. Every fourth will have diabetes. And six out of 10 will have more than one chronic condition. By 2015, there will be 600,000 hip replacements and 1.4 million knee replacements needed.[1] Understanding these consumers will be crucial.

"I make a new choice every time," a patient once told me. Even though she has a good relationship with one provider, she starts her search anew every time she needs hospital care. It might be a little more difficult to market to a boomer. Or will it?

Who are they?

Many marketers try to categorize and define the boomer population, but one size does not fit all. Even marketing experts and consultancies segment this market in various ways. From a demographic standpoint, first ask some qualifying questions.

For example, how is the age composition of your markets changing? Traditional college towns may see an influx of boomer retirees who place a premium on life-long learning. What about the marital status of the boomers in your market? One-third of boomers (23 million) are single. They don't have children or a deep support network to care for them as they age. How will the community step in, and what role will hospitals play?

Demographics are a start, but we need to know more. With boomers, the emphasis is not so much on age as it is on life stage. According to The Boomer Project *(www.boomerproject.com)*, this demographic could be parents, retirees, caregivers, empty nesters, entrepreneurs, grandparents, or some combination thereof. Grandparents are one of the largest and most powerful consumer segments in the United

States today. Factor that into your community relations efforts. Sponsoring the local soccer team is a good way to show that your hospital is a good citizen. With grandmothers and grandfathers showing up to root on their little stars, these community activities take on a whole new strategic importance.

Reaching out to boomers

Members of this consumer segment are absolutely interested in their health. Robin Wight, chair of WCRS, a well-known UK advertising agency, may have defined boomers best: "It is a young mind, in an aging body, with a maturing wallet." Before the 2008 stock market crash, this last comment was true.

Even though boomers want to stay out of the hospital, they will inevitably need care. You must create tipping points that will convince people to choose your organization and your physicians.

Here are some strategies:

- **Engagement.** Boomers like one-to-one communication. They like to be considered a VIP. So engage them. Put them on advisory boards to help you craft your marketing. You could start with orthopedics or neurosurgery as a pilot and expand to other areas of the hospital. Give identified influencers sneak previews and access to information. Make them privy to the destination center development plans well before others.

- **Cause marketing.** According to Focalyst, a research arm of AARP that focuses on boomers, 70% of boomers say they have a responsibility to

Orthopedics and Spine

make the world a better place. Causes affect philanthropy. What cause can you adopt with your boomer market? Take the lead. And don't forget to involve complementary organizations and those that target boomers but don't compete with you.

- **Give to get.** Some hospitals offer a free in-home assessment for postsurgical patients so that when they come home, they will be able to recuperate in the best environment possible. Talk about service after the sale. Before the hip or knee replacement, send a team to the patient's home to assess the environment and make the needed changes for a quality recovery. That reflects well on you and their PCPs.

The message for the 50-plus crowd

Any good marketing campaign starts with the message. Here is what resonates:

- **Youthful, not young.** Older people make decisions based on the age they feel rather than the age they are. According to The Boomer Project, 50-year-olds see themselves as 12 years younger than their chronological age. Gear your message and images accordingly. Single older women are important images and reflect the marketplace.

- **Forward-looking, not nostalgic.** Boomers are moving ahead, not looking behind. Commercials featuring Dennis Hopper recalling the 1960s play only so far. They have much of their lives ahead of them, with a lot of plans and ideas for how to spend that time. Show them how they'll spend more of that time enjoying a great quality of life after you take care of them.

- **Humorous, not calamitous.** Humor is powerful, but it's also difficult to get right. Remember, boomers span many years and have a range of values, outlooks, and frames of reference. Don't scare them or make them feel inadequate.

- **Positive, not negative.** Research shows that older consumers have trained their brains to ignore negative images or ideas. Be uplifting.

- **Educational, not preachy.** Give boomers the tools to understand why your service is better, and give them the opportunity to make their own choices. Give them easy-to-consume chunks of information. They can't be told; they have to be led subtly.

- **Honest, not slick.** Provide honest and literate messages. When marketing to boomers, education works much better than promotion and sales.

- **Right-brained, not left.** As people age, emotions, hunches, feelings, possibilities, probabilities, and life experiences play a larger role. Tell a story. Use testimonials. Aim inwardly. They might connect with a compelling photograph that conjures up certain emotions and feelings. Once you grab them emotionally, be prepared to give the facts so they can make their own decisions. Realize more is not always better.

- **Independent, not dependent.** Use the language of independence. Give them the tools to make decisions.

- **Multimodal, not single-minded.** Boomers are still traditionalists, but they also use technology. About half subscribe to newspapers and two-thirds

 Orthopedics and Spine

read the Sunday paper. Then again, 75% have cell phones and 11% have iPods. In people over age 50, 80% feel that computers are easy to use and one in four spend more time on their PC than watching TV.

Return on Investment

So how do you know if your marketing is working? Marketing has been murky for many years when it comes to return on investment. To some degree, it's always going to be difficult to pinpoint the cause and effect. Smart marketers use data to target customers. And when you target them, you include a call to action. It sounds logical, yet many hospitals do not do this. If you send out a direct-mail piece, you need to code it so you know what campaign generated it. Create a specific phone number to call or Web site to visit to track results. As real prospect names surface, add them to your customer relationship management database and track them through the system.

Summary

Marketing is important and includes many components:

- A thorough and systematic approach to understanding who your customers are and what they want and need

- Understanding whether your service offerings meet these needs

- Informing leadership where the gaps are and how to narrow them

- Crafting messages that will make your customers aware of how you are meeting their needs

- Differentiating yourself so that your services are sought rather than sold

Build your destination center of superior performance around the needs of your customers. They in turn will tell the world. This is marketing at its best.

Endnote

1. Victoria Stagg Elliot, "Hip, knee replacement surgery rates skyrocket over 7 years," *American Medical News*, *www.ama-assn.org/amednews/2008/05/05/hlsb0505.htm* (accessed June 24, 2009).

Service Line Subspecialties in Action

Contributing writers: Thomas Graham, MD, Bill Munley, MBA, Patrick Vega, MS, Mary Ann Sweeney, PT

Part of the appeal of developing orthopedic service lines is the plethora of possibilities for subspecialty programs. This chapter is divided into two sections. The first discusses inpatient programs, such as total joint replacement, spine, and fracture care. The second covers outpatient care, such as outpatient spine, sports medicine, foot and ankle, and hand surgery.

The keys to successfully assessing, designing, implementing, managing, marketing, and sustaining these centers are discussed in the previous chapters of this book. Here we'll focus on what makes each subspecialty unique and provide case studies from which we can all learn.

Part 1: Inpatient Programs

Joint and Spine

The core of every musculoskeletal destination center is the implementation of extraordinary inpatient programs for joint and spine patients. The traditional inpatient care model for joint and spine patients has often resulted in mediocre patient experiences, surgeon dissatisfaction, and low margins. Few hospitals have implemented focused joint and spine programs led by surgeons. Even fewer hospitals and surgeons measure their results post-intervention or have robust metrics to support thoughtful clinical and operational management decisions.

The development of destination inpatient centers for joint and spine surgery will be essential in the future to care for patients requiring these procedures. No hospital is too small to develop an excellent, efficient, and patient-centric joint or spine program. Although it is not easy, a high-quality joint and spine center can be implemented within a six-month period. Leadership and vision are needed, as is collaboration among surgeons, administration, and staff members. The model will not only change joint and spine replacement surgery, but it will change the entire culture of the hospital.

The time is right. Baby boomers are approaching age 65. They have been more active than any previous generation, thus putting more stress on their backs, knees, and hips. Many of these boomers have or will develop arthritis and need care, including total joint replacement (TJR) surgery and spine surgery. The forecast is that by 2030:

- Hip replacements will increase from 225,000 to 600,000

- Knee replacements will increase from 430,000 to 1,400,000

- Spine cases, both inpatient and outpatient, will continue to increase at double-digit levels

Despite these astounding numbers, not every hospital or surgeon will benefit. Highly educated patients will look for hospitals and surgeons that have made a commitment to care for these conditions. This commitment will include dedicated facilities and staff members as well as programs that improve their experience. They will look for hospitals and surgeons who measure and share results.

Many hospitals struggle to make TJR profitable. More than half of the patients are of Medicare age, and the reimbursement is quite low. Every total joint patient needs an operating room (OR), an implant, and usually a hospital stay. Most hospital ORs are expensive and inefficient. Implants can consume a large percentage of the reimbursement. Surgeons traditionally do not like to change implants or get involved in price negotiations.

Hospital care is often costly, inefficiently managed, and not service-oriented. Hospitals that don't measure what matters and fail to create the right management structures will be at a huge disadvantage clinically and financially. Without the right data in the hands of those that can make the most difference (physicians and staff members), change will be painfully slow. Costs will continue to be higher than necessary, and clinical improvements will not be realized quickly across the entire patient population.

A significant shortage of joint surgeons is expected going forward. Fewer and fewer orthopedic surgeons are specializing in TJR because reimbursement is low and the effort and risk are quite high. There are even fewer spine surgeons. In fact, neurosurgeons are increasingly the only surgeons performing spine surgery at many hospitals, and neurosurgeons are even more difficult to recruit than orthopedic surgeons. Therefore, it is essential to develop a center that is attractive not only to patients, but to surgeons as well. One of the main issues for surgeons is OR efficiency and availability. Providing efficiencies that will allow a surgeon to perform twice as many surgeries in one day is a huge satisfier.

To create an advantage for all stakeholders, destination joint and spine programs must address all of these issues. These inpatient programs must deliver such a unique and wonderful experience for patients that they will rave about you incessantly. They must create and support such an experience for physicians that they wouldn't want their patients anywhere else. The same goes for nurses and other staff members. The program must be profitable so that the hospital can afford to invest in it. This results in a spirit of cooperation between joint and spine surgeons and the hospital and often becomes a model for other services to emulate.

Joints vs. spine

I put joint and spine inpatient programs into one section because they have so much in common. Most are elective. Most require an inpatient stay. Most candidates are mature adults who are not in peak physical condition.

There are differences, however. In joint replacement surgery, 90% or more of the patients require either a hip or knee replacement, with a few shoulders and ankles.

Most of them are over age 60. Many are over 80. They are often retired. They usually have had the problem for years and can be scheduled quite far in advance. After surgery, a two- or three-day stay is usually required.

In spine, there are a wide variety of procedures performed in both the cervical and lumbar region. The age range is more diverse. Most patients are working. Their hospital stay after the procedure ranges from a few hours (outpatient) to three days. Some patients have had the problem for years, but many are semi-elective, quite acute, or occasionally urgent. Despite these differences, the fundamentals of creating inpatient joint and spine centers are similar. In fact, many hospitals that perform fewer than 300 annual joint and spine procedures implement them as one inpatient program. When volumes exceed this number, they are usually separate programs.

The key elements are similar for both programs and are included in other sections of this book. They are as follows:

- The patient-centric care model:

    - Community

    - Primary care

    - Specialists

    - Preoperative preparation

    - Operative care

- Hospital care

- Postoperative care

- Outcomes and management

• The core elements of excellence:

- The right people

- Right structure

- Effective processes

- Excellent results

• Measuring what matters:

- Functional outcomes (did the procedure meet or exceed the patient's expectations six months or more after being performed?)

- Clinical, operational, financial, and patient experience

• Managing from metrics:

- Leadership team

- Performance improvement team

- Effective long-term marketing:

  - Community service

  - Primary care

  - Word of mouth

Creating a comprehensive destination center that has all the elements noted previously can lead to spectacular results. Consider a sampling of the results reported by hospitals that have created this model:

- Patient satisfaction percentile scores rising from 26th to 99th

- Length of stay (LOS) reductions of 30% to 50%

- Contribution margins increased by 100%

- Cost reductions of more than $1 million

- Reduction in vendors from eight to three

- Turnover times reduced from 45 to 11 minutes

- Service-line market share doubling the hospital market share

- Volume growth of 30% or more

- Rate of patients going directly home after surgery reaching 90% or higher

Joint/spine center case studies

Important lessons can be gleaned from each of the following case studies.

1. Lubbock, TX, 995-bed hospital

A comparison was made between two control groups receiving joint surgery from the same five surgeons. Between October 2005 and June 2008, 653 consecutive patients were admitted for hip and knee replacement surgeries. The following results compare the cases of the 248 patients admitted during the 13 months prior to the implementation of the destination total joint center/standardized protocols with the results of 405 patients admitted during the first 19 months of service-line implementation.

The destination center group of patients benefited in the following ways:

- Decrease in LOS from 4.19 to 3 days

- Overall pain scores decreased by 38%

- Ambulation increased by 481%

- Range of motion increased by 57%

2. Flagstaff, AZ, 250-bed community hospital

Surgeon-hospital relations were already strong at this 250-bed community hospital; however, service-line focus and development had not been part of the hospital's culture. New facilities and state-of-the-art technology had failed to substantially increase volume, and future growth was at risk due to the threat of a planned opening of a local, surgeon-owned ambulatory surgery center (ASC).

After executing the principles outlined in this book, the service line experienced the following results within the first year:

- Volume increase of 16%

- LOS reduced by 20%, saving $350,000 in year one

- 16% increase in the number of patients being discharged home after surgery

3. Knoxville, TN, 250-bed community hospital

Although joint replacement volume was already high, surgeon relationships with the hospital were not optimal. In addition, two competing hospital systems in town were contemplating the opening of a new joint replacement unit, putting the hospital at risk of losing patients and surgeons.

During the first year:

- Patient satisfaction scores averaged in the 99th percentile

- The joint unit became the third highest performing unit in the health system

- Total distance ambulated by postop day three averaged 2,000 ft.

- Case volume grew 15%

- Average LOS decreased from 4.6 days to 3.1 days

4. Annapolis, MD, 260-bed community hospital

After a joint program was implemented in 1996, a spine program was created in 1998 using the same principles. At the time the second program was added, there were two orthopedic surgeons and two neurosurgeons doing spine surgery.

During the first year:

- The volume tripled

- LOS and cost were significantly lower than state averages

- Spine became one of top three profit centers in the hospital

- The number of spine surgeons doubled, with equal numbers in spine and neurosurgery

5. University Hospital, Maastricht, the Netherlands

Of 160 consecutive patients, 80 were randomly selected to be cared for in a joint program and 80 in the traditional way.

During year one, the joint recovery program experienced:

- More than a 50% reduction in LOS

- Significant average cost saving per patient:

    - $1,261 in the total hip replacement group

    - $3,336 in the total knee replacement group

- Significantly higher functional level and quality of life vs. traditional care patients

The development of destination inpatient centers in joint and spine are beneficial for all stakeholders. Patient, physician, and staff satisfaction will rise dramatically. Costs will decrease, and profitability will rise. Results can be tracked and changes made based on this information. You will begin to brand and differentiate yourself. A spirit of collaboration will ensue, and this will have an effect on your entire organization. You will be well positioned for the changes we are about to experience in healthcare. In fact, you will be helping to lead those changes.

Geriatric Fracture Centers

Most hospitals are not level-one trauma centers, although nearly all of them treat fractures. Geriatric fractures make up a significant number of the fractures that require hospitalization. This section discusses a geriatric fracture program; however, the principles outlined here can be extended to the care of any fracture that needs hospital admission.

Unlike many joint and spine procedures, fractures are never elective. Although it may be easier to create programs and consistency in elective surgery, it is no less important to do so with nonelective surgery. Implementing a comprehensive geriatric fracture care program can be cost-effective, is the right thing to do, and can help brand you. A society is measured by the way it treats its elderly, which will one day include you.

Consider the epidemiology of hip fractures. 350,000 currently occur per year, and the incidence is increasing: The number is estimated to grow to 650,000 by 2050. The United States spends about $18 billion per year on fragility fractures. They occur most often in people over age 80, and 80% of the fractures occur in females. Women have a one in seven lifetime chance of suffering a hip fracture.

The main risk factor for geriatric hip fracture is osteoporosis. Other risk factors include dementia, unstable gait, poor muscle strength, poor vision, neurological disease, and poor nutrition.

Hip fracture surgeries are usually performed by on-call general orthopedists who perform a handful of these cases per year. We see fewer and fewer orthopedists interested in taking call and performing this surgery. In addition, fracture patients are often deconditioned prior to surgery. Caregivers at home are lacking. You can see what a challenge these patients and our hospitals are up against.

Consider these characteristics about mainstream fracture care:

- 30%–50% of hip fracture patients will die in the first 12 months post-injury

- The postoperative delirium rate approaches 80%

- Pneumonia, urinary tract infections, and wound infections are common complications

- Deep vein thrombosis (DVT) is common unless anticoagulation therapy is used postoperatively

- Hip fractures are usually a financial loser for hospitals

Despite these challenges, patients who are successfully returned to their pre-injury levels of activity have a 70%–80% chance of resuming independent living.

Every hospital that treats fractures, especially hip fractures, should create a geriatric fracture center. The mission should be to speed recovery time in osteoporotic hip fracture patients, initiate osteoporosis education and treatment, prevent future fractures in this high-risk population, and educate the public in prevention. Fracture patients over age 45 with low-velocity injuries who are admitted should be considered for the inpatient geriatric fracture program.

The goals of such a program are to:

- Promptly identify and reduce surgical risk factors

- Quickly get the patient to surgery and recovery

- Prevent a second fracture

- Identify existing bone density and nutritional deficiencies

- Initiate vitamin D and calcium supplementation

- Provide patient and family education

- Initiate secondary osteoporosis workup (endocrinology consult) if necessary

- Coordinate a bone treatment plan with the appropriate primary care physician (PCP)

- Coordinate a bone treatment plan with the appropriate physical therapist

- Return quality of life as quickly as possible

- Provide cost-effective care

- Measure appropriate outcomes

Hospitals should also consider creating an outpatient program for preventing second fractures in patients age 45 or older with osteoporotic fractures of the wrist, proximal humerus, spine, and hip. The goals of such programs are to provide public education and support regarding fracture care and prevention.

Fracture care case study

The following case study was contributed by William E. Munley, vice president of orthopedics and professional services at Bon Secours St. Francis Health System in Greenville, SC. It focuses on fracture care, but the lessons learned can be applied to any orthopedic subspecialty.

HOW WAS CARE BEING DELIVERED
IN OUR INSTITUTION (AND PERHAPS YOURS)?

This hypothetical story takes place in 2005 and involves a patient who could be any-one's mother or grandmother. She is a 76-year-old independent ambulator and lives at home alone. She drives herself to church, visits friends, and does her own shop-ping. When she falls at home and fractures her hip, she calls an ambulance and is transported by emergency medical services (EMS) to the emergency department (ED) at St. Francis Hospital Downtown.

Once in the ED, she is triaged as nonurgent, a Foley catheter is placed, and narcotics are started for pain control. X-rays and labs are obtained, and she spends the next seven hours in the ED.

She is admitted by an on-call orthopedist over the telephone and transferred to a standard room on the orthopedic floor. Buck's traction is applied and medical con-sults are ordered. An extensive preop medical workup is done over the next 48 hours, after which she is finally cleared for surgery and placed on a waiting list as nonurgent. No social worker will contact her until after her surgery.

Surgery is completed at 11:00 the next evening after the patient was bumped for more urgent cases. The procedure is performed by an on-call hospital OR team, and the fracture is finally stabilized about 72 hours after the injury.

Postop delirium occurs and lasts 48 hours. There is little if any physical therapy (PT) during this time, and the Foley catheter is left in place. The family is anxious about the patient's altered mental status.

The postoperative course continues with slow progress in physical and occupational therapy, and the therapy is performed by staff members with little geriatric experience.

HOW WAS CARE BEING DELIVERED
IN OUR INSTITUTION (AND PERHAPS YOURS)? (CONT.)

A urinary tract infection (UTI) develops due to extended use of the catheter, requiring antibiotics. The family is anxious about what to do next, so a social worker begins to explain options.

The patient is finally discharged and transferred to an inpatient rehabilitation facility on postop day seven. She is discharged on antibiotics for the UTI as well as narcotic pain medicines. She has been given no medication for osteoporosis.

She eventually gets transferred to long-term care, and expires four months after surgery, having never returned to her home.

We did not know any better but to accept this kind of result. In fact, if my own 80-year-old mother went through all of this, I would have accepted the outcome as normal. Today, I realize that a geriatric fracture care program may have resulted in a different outcome.

A call to arms

In late 2005, we finally had a "call to arms." Our main orthopedic trauma surgeon, Dr. Michael O'Boyle, called me excitedly to discuss a new geriatric fracture program. As a vice president of a health system, my first thought was, "Why is my high-powered orthopedic trauma surgeon so interested in one of the least glamorous procedures in all of orthopedics?" However, I really respected Dr. O'Boyle's opinion.

Vision and goals

The first step was to develop a concise business plan. We started with a vision statement, which said: "The development of a Geriatric Long Bone/Hip Fracture Center of Excellence would allow St. Francis Hospital to strategically position itself in the local market and nearby communities as the geriatric orthopedic center of choice.

HOW WAS CARE BEING DELIVERED
IN OUR INSTITUTION (AND PERHAPS YOURS)? (CONT.)

The program would utilize a multidisciplinary, multispecialty team approach to facilitate market share growth and quality outcomes."

We projected that such a program would either feed into or be fed by seminars and education programs, balance master referrals, hip/long bone fractures, inpatient rehabilitation admissions, osteoporosis screenings, outpatient rehab, and/or degenerative surgical spine cases. In fact, we later developed an osteoporosis program as a direct result of developing the geriatric fracture center.

We were also very aggressive in developing the following programmatic goals to:

- Provide education for bone health and injury prevention

- Offer screenings for osteoporosis

- Transition patients from the ED to the nursing floor within 4.5 hours

- Transition patients from the ED to surgery within 12–24 hours

- Reduce pain levels

- Reduce LOS to 5.5 days or fewer

- Enhance functional outcomes

- Reduce long-term nursing home placements

- Reduce mortality in the first year following fractures

- Increase patient satisfaction scores

> **HOW WAS CARE BEING DELIVERED**
> **IN OUR INSTITUTION (AND PERHAPS YOURS)? (CONT.)**
>
> • Maintain our five-star HealthGrades quality rating for hip fracture repair
>
> • Increase volume of fracture patients
>
> Officially, we rolled out the program in January 2007. This was the first program of its kind in South Carolina. We developed our geriatric fracture center program menu for success based on various operational changes, which included the addition of key personnel plus formalized administrative support.
>
> First, it was very easy to name our medical director/physician champion, as Dr. O'Boyle had shown such passion for this program and its patients. He enthusiastically accepted.
>
> Second, we hired 1.5 fracture center coordinators to act as navigators for the program. They not only act as facilitators internally, but also serve as external liaisons with area nursing homes, providing follow-up care to our patients and follow-up education to the nursing home staff. They are on-call 24 hours a day, seven days a week, to help follow patients' progress from the time they reach the ED until 90 days post-discharge.
>
> The development of the multidisciplinary team was also critical. First, we identified EMS as a key member of our team. These personnel care what happens to their patients, and they can have some influence as to what hospital the patient chooses. Next, we selected key physicians from the ED, hospitalist group, anesthesia, physical medicine and rehabilitation, medical staff services, and of course, orthopedics. Internally, we selected team members from imaging and lab, the OR, therapy, the nursing unit, case management and discharge planning, marketing and planning, and administration. Representatives from administration included four vice presidents,

HOW WAS CARE BEING DELIVERED
IN OUR INSTITUTION (AND PERHAPS YOURS)? (CONT.)

three administrative directors, and multiple department heads. We also included our own inpatient rehab center staff and representatives from various nursing homes on the team. Finally, we named patients and family as part of the team.

A regular meeting schedule for this multidisciplinary team is imperative. We hold monthly or bimonthly clinical subcommittee meetings on the floor. We also hold monthly geriatric fracture center meetings of the full committee, which can sometimes involve up to 30 people. At least five case studies are discussed at these monthly meetings, split between success stories and those cases where something in the process could be improved. This case study discussion serves as a mode of continuing education for the physicians and staff members. It also allows for continuous process improvement.

A process to benefit all

We created a streamlined evaluation and admission process that makes the job of the ED physicians a little easier. New ED orders were developed, enabling the physician to fast-track lab and imaging studies. Once the patient is identified as a hip fracture patient, the fracture center coordinator and hospitalist are notified.

The fracture center coordinator notifies the orthopedist on call and prepares the nursing floor for the admission process. The hospitalist stabilizes the patient and admits to the orthopedic floor. Standardized orders are implemented and the clinical pathway is initiated.

This changes the flow of the patient's progress considerably. The old method had the orthopedist as the admitting physician who also did the surgery and follow-up patient care until discharge. Now it is the hospitalist who admits, clears the patient medically, and prepares him or her for the OR within 12–24 hours of arrival in the ED.

HOW WAS CARE BEING DELIVERED
IN OUR INSTITUTION (AND PERHAPS YOURS)? (CONT.)

Our administration is thoroughly convinced that this process is best practice. There-fore, all orthopedists performing hip fracture surgery must sign a letter of agreement stating that they will abide by the established protocols. The most important of these protocols are getting the patient to the OR within 12–24 hours and utilizing the cor-rect order sets.

OR time is reserved five days a week for these patients. If the patient arrives in the ED and we can finish the case by 9:00 that evening, we will perform the surgery. If not, the surgery will be performed first thing the next morning. The specialized staff in the OR enhances efficiency. Under this setup, Dr. O'Boyle frequently can do a "skin to skin" case in less than 20 minutes.

To give the unit its own identity, we dedicated seven beds on our orthopedic floor to the geriatric fracture center. Because our seventh-floor orthopedic unit was under-going a facelift anyway, we were able to custom design some items in the patient rooms. With the volume of hip fracture patients being unpredictable, we allow over-flow of other patients into these rooms, but we always keep at least two rooms open for geriatric fractures.

Because the census is unpredictable and it is only a seven-bed unit housing 280 patients per year, we use specially trained—rather than exclusively dedicated—staff members throughout the OR, nursing unit, discharge planning, and therapy depart-ments. Although this staff may treat other patients in the hospital, its primary respon-sibility is dealing with the geriatric fracture patients. The early morning OR staff can set up and turn over the room very quickly, helping the surgeon's efficiency. The floor nurses initiate and carry out the clinical pathway, and therapists initiate very aggres-sive therapy early in the process. Likewise, our discharge planners meet with patients and/or families on day one. Other patient/family education also begins on day one

 Orthopedics and Spine

HOW WAS CARE BEING DELIVERED
IN OUR INSTITUTION (AND PERHAPS YOURS)? (CONT.)

because we want their active participation in the decision-making process even before surgery, if possible.

Measuring and managing

We also developed dashboards to establish baselines, measure against published and self-established benchmarks, and monitor our progress. We tried to develop our dashboards around four areas: quality, service and satisfaction, volume, and cost. We also wanted to establish real outcome measures in addition to the normal compliance measures that are seen on most dashboards.

The items monitored under the quality section of the dashboard include percentages of mortality rates one year postop; infections; patients coming to us from independent living vs. nursing homes; patients from independent living that returned to their former living arrangement and/or maintain independent living postop; patients transferred to our inpatient rehab center; percentage of time that the fracture care coordinator was called by ED upon the fracture admission; time between ED arrival to surgery in less than 12 hours (our stretch goal); time between ED arrival to surgery in less than 24 hours; time between ED arrival to nursing floor in less than 4.5 hours; and clinical pathway utilization initiated by the floor nurses. We also measure the percentile of excellent rankings in our patient callback survey, set quarterly goals for the number of seminars and/or screenings in the community, and monitor our HealthGrades rankings.

On the cost side, we measure direct cost per case and LOS broken down by diagnosis-related groups (DRG) 469, 470, 480, 481, and 482. These figures are compared against those of the previous two to four fiscal years and are then compared against our current goal. We also established goals and monitor results for volumes in the same way.

HOW WAS CARE BEING DELIVERED
IN OUR INSTITUTION (AND PERHAPS YOURS)? (CONT.)

In addition, each surgeon participating in our program is monitored on our physician dashboard and receives monthly as well as year-to-date results. Items on this dashboard include average LOS equal to or less than five days; patients to the OR within 24 hours from ED arrival; patients to the OR within 12 hours from ED arrival (our stretch goal); order sets compliance; DVT protocol compliance; percentage of patients with postop delirium; percentage of patients with pain scores of less than three at discharge; patient/family satisfaction scores of five (excellent); and evidence of patient/family education. If a surgeon falls off of any one of these areas on the dashboard two months in a row, our vice president of medical staff services contacts him or her for an explanation.

Marketing

After these operational and programmatic changes were implemented, we embarked on our marketing efforts to get the word out. We have a good relationship with EMS and continue to nurture our partnership. Our community outreach goals are accomplished by providing seminars and educational sessions to churches, senior centers, assisted living centers, and other public venues. Our staff provides inservices to area nursing homes, and the geriatric fracture center coordinators spend at least two days per week in the nursing homes providing administrative liaison work and follow-up care for the patients.

We developed our osteoporosis program as a spin-off of the geriatric fracture center to function as a mutual feeding mechanism into fracture care and other programs. We developed collateral materials, such as brochures with a detachable pocket/purse card that reads, "Take Me to St. Francis." We also provide St. Francis night lights to all of our fracture patients. The word spread quickly among the media, and we were featured in newspaper articles, television news briefs, and television shows.

HOW WAS CARE BEING DELIVERED
IN OUR INSTITUTION (AND PERHAPS YOURS)? (CONT.)

What fracture care looks like today

So what did all these changes mean to the next 76-year-old female who fell and broke her hip? In 2008, when a similar patient falls at home, she will still be taken by ambulance to the ED. But that's where the similarities end.

In the ED, she's triaged as a priority probable hip fracture. The geriatric fracture center coordinator is immediately notified, as is the hospitalist to admit the patient. The care coordinator will contact the orthopedist on call. Standardized orders are implemented, a catheter is placed, narcotics are started for pain control, and she spends less than four hours in the ED.

She is transferred to a specialized room on the seventh-floor orthopedic unit in the geriatric fracture center (or even directly to the OR). Her preop process goes smoothly, and she is cleared for surgery within six hours of admission. A social worker meets with her and her family, and patient/family education is initiated. She is scheduled for surgery in a dedicated fracture time slot in the OR.

Surgery is completed within 12–24 hours of the injury and is performed by a dedicated hip fracture team.

Back on the floor, her postoperative course begins. There is no delay in PT because of delirium, and there is less reliance on narcotics for pain control. A Foley catheter is removed on postop day one. Her family is now actively involved in her rehab and postoperative planning.

The patient is ambulating on postop day one with specially trained therapists. The social worker and rehabilitation physician are working with the patient and her family on short-term rehab placement after discharge. She is transferred either to

---

**HOW WAS CARE BEING DELIVERED
IN OUR INSTITUTION (AND PERHAPS YOURS)? (CONT.)**

the inpatient rehab center (IRC) or a select skilled nursing facility (SNF) on postop day three or four. She is discharged from acute care with no narcotic pain medicine, and osteoporosis treatment is initiated with a follow-up bone density test ordered.

She spends two to four weeks in the IRC or SNF, with the geriatric fracture coordinator visiting her and her family for continuing education as well as providing information to the orthopedist regarding her progress and/or complications. She returns home to independent living within six weeks. She is now on osteoporosis medications, fall precautions, and an exercise program to minimize the risk of another fragility fracture. She is driving herself to church again.

Results by the numbers
Before we started the program, our LOS for this DRG was 7.29 days. Patients sometimes waited up to four days in the hospital before their surgery was performed. We have seen phenomenal outcomes in the two years of the program:

- ED to floor time has decreased from 6 hours to 3.9 hours on average

- ED to incision time has decreased from 68.7 hours to 17 hours on average.

- Average LOS has decreased from 7.3 days to less than 4 days

- Implant costs have decreased due to standardization

- OR costs have decreased due to specialized teams and time slots

- The contribution margin has demonstrated a $2,000 per-case positive turnaround

- Almost 80% of our patients who come to us from independent living return to their former living arrangements or other independent living

HOW WAS CARE BEING DELIVERED
IN OUR INSTITUTION (AND PERHAPS YOURS)? (CONT.)

- The mortality rate one-year postop is beginning to creep under 20%

- Postoperative delirium rates are less than 4%

- Infection rates are less than 1%

- Patient satisfaction is 100%

- We remain at five stars in hip fracture repair through the 2009 HealthGrades report

And most importantly, we are able to claim and live by the phrase, "We move patients to the next phase of their life, before the competition even puts them under the knife!"

Part II: Outpatient Programs

Outpatient Spine Care

Nearly every hospital, from the community hospital to the large academic facility, provides some form of spine care: imaging, surgery, pain management, and PT. Nationally, back and neck pain represent the second most common reason patients see a doctor, with 13.7 million people visiting physician offices for back pain each year. Chronic back pain accounts for 15% of all sick leaves and is the leading cause of adult disability. Approximately 85%–90% of back pain patients can be treated effectively with nonoperative interventions, such as PT or pain medications.

Spine also remains one of the more favorably reimbursed specialties. For hospitals and physician practices, a destination spine center represents a significant growth opportunity in terms of program development, increased market share, and profitability. New surgical technologies for the spine have enabled this market to experience over 10% growth per year during the past decade. Spine surgical procedures represent a significant portion of neurosurgical and orthopedic surgery and will drive significant future growth in neurosciences and orthopedics.

Although the majority of spine surgery is currently performed within hospital walls, improved pain management, minimally invasive surgical techniques, and new device technologies will accelerate the steerage of certain types of surgical cases to ASCs.

Unique challenges

Spine care is less straightforward than other subspecialties because its diagnostic and treatment options are so diverse. Consider the following factors:

- **A wide variety of nonsurgical treatments:** rest, medications, PT, manipulation, massage, Reiki, epidural steroid injections, nerve blocks, electrical stimulation, acupuncture, or a combination of modalities.

- **A wide variety of surgical procedures:** neck and back posterior fusions, anterior fusions, decompressions, and open and minimally invasive techniques.

- **Lack of consensus on best practices.** Individual physicians still define best practice. It is not uncommon for surgeons to offer varying explanations and recommendations.

- **Individual providers don't measure outcomes.** Although "outcomes" are routinely referenced, there is a dearth of data by individual physicians, leading to a perception among payers, physicians, and patients that the procedures are not effective.

- **Many nonsurgical patients are treated by surgeons.** Due to lack of triage protocols and desire to see neurosurgeons and orthopedists, it is not uncommon for surgeons to treat a disproportionate percentage of nonsurgical patients.

- **Access issues.** Back pain is disabling, making it difficult for sufferers to access care. Many end up in emergency rooms when they can no longer bear the discomfort.

- Multiple nonoperative spine care providers:

  - Neurosurgery

  - Orthopedics

  - Primary care

  - Neurology

  - Physiatry

  - Anesthesia/pain

  - Chiropractic

  - PT

  - Alternative, complementary, and integrative medicine, such as Reiki, acupuncture, acupressure, and healing touch

  - "Spinologist" is a term recently coined by a large academic spine program to describe a spine specialist who is charged with initial evaluations and determining triage, essentially serving as a gatekeeper and directing to providers of care

- Overlapping surgical specialists, particularly neurosurgery and orthopedics. The first successful lumbar discectomy was carried out at Massachusetts General Hospital in Boston by Dr. William Mixter, a neurosurgeon, and Dr. Joseph Barr, an orthopedic surgeon. This sharing of spine surgery continues today. Spine surgery is taught in both orthopedic and neurosurgical training programs. In many institutions, the two specialties work closely together. In others, they act more like competitors.

- **High competition for ancillaries.** Ancillary revenues are significant, but there is competition from community imaging centers, outpatient rehabilitation, and outpatient surgery centers for pain management. It is likely that hospitals need a robust intake and triage system, supported by navigation, if they expect to capture this revenue.

Access and navigation

As a result of these challenges, the principles of patient-centric care and core elements of excellence apply not only to inpatient programs, but outpatient ones as well. Although the concept of navigation is described in Chapter 5, the access issues particular to spine patients warrant further explanation on guiding these patients through the continuum of care.

It is not uncommon for patients seeking care for back and neck pain to report a lengthy and unsatisfying process of getting to the right provider and finding relief. Frequently, the first referral is made by a PCP to a surgeon for consultation—often with a four- to eight-week wait for an appointment. With the vast majority of patients needing nonsurgical care, they are understandably frustrated by long waits and long drives for specialist consults, only to be told they're not surgical candidates, need further diagnostic tests, or need to see a different specialist. Consulting surgeons are likewise frustrated that so many of these patients are nonsurgical and could have been referred to other specialists for nonoperative care.

With exhausting caseloads, it's challenging for PCPs to refer their patients to the most appropriate specialist or order the most appropriate diagnostic tests. When referral is required, surgeons are often selected because of their breadth of knowledge about nonsurgical and surgical care. PCPs, like their patients, are often frustrated by access issues.

Because of the acute pain, disability, and loss of function associated with back pain, consumers will seek the most visible, accessible, and responsive provider, regardless of provider outcomes and clinical appropriateness of treatments. This predictable behavior is cautionary for both patient and spine specialist; patients may engage in treatments that are not effective, and providers may receive patients better served by a colleague in another spine subspecialty.

Due to the often disabling nature of back pain and its effect on social and professional life, psychosocial comorbidities (e.g., depression, anxiety, chronic pain, and high-dose narcotic use) are more prevalent among spine patients. Additionally, a significant percentage of spine care patients have filed workers' compensation claims, which can add complexity to care due to claimant and defendant legal issues, opposing medical opinions, and the adversarial nature of the claims process.

In nearly every community, the current system of intake, triage, and referral (ITR) resides exclusively in the respective physician offices. Each has its own protocols and procedures for accepting and treating referrals from medical professionals and self-referred patients. Physicians often characterize the coordination of access, evaluation, and treatment as haphazard and poorly coordinated. It is both notable and encouraging that many medical staff and spine specialists recognize both the need and opportunities to improve service to medical professionals and self-referred patients.

The most effective antidote to these challenges is a comprehensive model of ITR that ensures patients are quickly directed to the most effective care modalities and to spine specialists most qualified to treat their unique symptoms. The goal of an effective ITR program is to create hospital and spine specialist ownership and sequential management of a typically inefficient, fragmented system.

A well-run ITR system supports and promotes the patient experience, spine specialists, referring physicians, and professional referral sources (e.g., workers' compensation, employer, and health plan). Specifically, an effective ITR:

- Places a priority on customer service to the patient and referring professional

- Provides expedited evaluation and treatment by the most clinically appropriate spine specialist

- Maximizes quality of face-to-face time with spine specialists

- Results in better clinical outcomes

- Stages the hospital to capture incremental ancillary procedures and revenues

In a fully developed ITR system, the first step is the referral from primary care, patient self-referral, and conceivably other spine specialists to an outpatient-based ITR system. This is often a hospital-supported activity. The ITR system's advantages include immediate response to callers, a centralized collection of clinical and demographic information, and administrative support for referring offices and self-referred patients.

The ITR algorithm in Figure 10.1 defines a methodology that has been collaboratively developed by affiliated spine specialists to determine the most appropriate first step in the course of care.

FIGURE 10.1

SAMPLE ALGORITHM

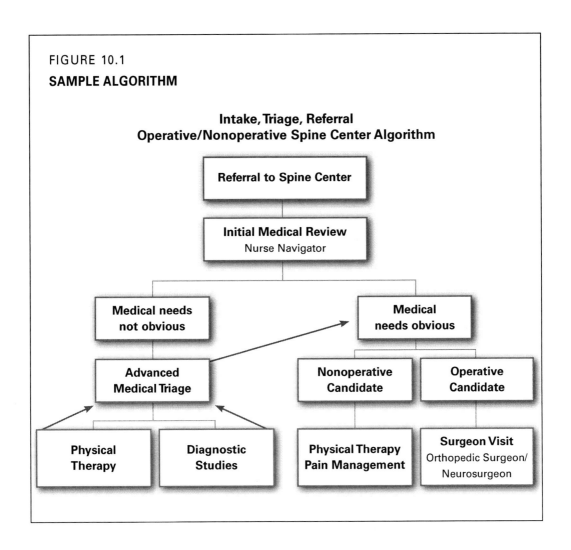

Intake, Triage, Referral
Operative/Nonoperative Spine Center Algorithm

Referral to Spine Center

Initial Medical Review
Nurse Navigator

Medical needs
not obvious

Medical
needs obvious

Advanced
Medical Triage

Nonoperative
Candidate

Operative
Candidate

Physical
Therapy

Diagnostic
Studies

Physical Therapy
Pain Management

Surgeon Visit
Orthopedic Surgeon/
Neurosurgeon

The critical role of advanced medical triage may be filled by surgeons, neurologists, physiatrists, nurse practitioners, and physician assistants. Individual institutions and their spine specialists will determine who plays this vital clinical role in patient flow and treatment. This person must be clinically respected, accessible, unbiased, and an excellent communicator to both patient and professional audiences.

Algorithms must be developed to assist with review and triage, as shown in Figure 10.2.

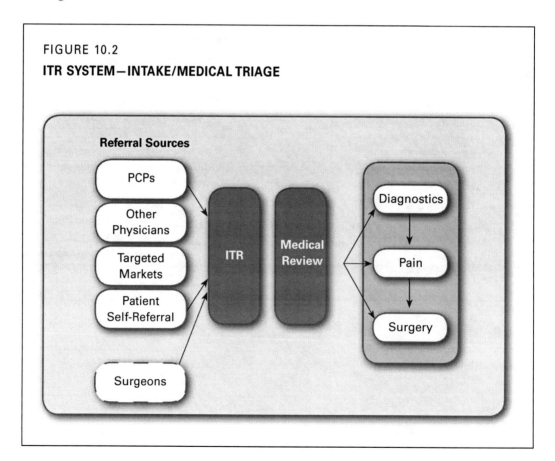

FIGURE 10.2

ITR SYSTEM—INTAKE/MEDICAL TRIAGE

The final sequence in an ITR process, shown in Figure 10.3, consists of making a clinically appropriate referral of the patient for surgical care.

FIGURE 10.3

ITR SYSTEM—FULL PROCESS

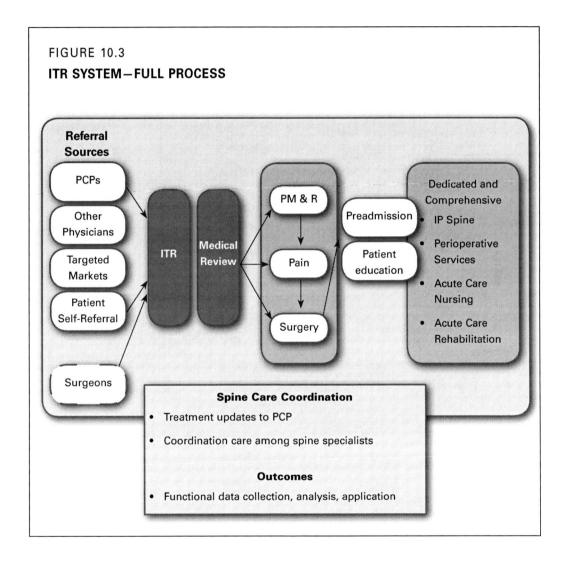

Although intake and referral is the critical first step, navigation and tracking is another important aspect of the ITR system. A navigator will provide care coordination and communication with all stakeholders.

To review the information in Chapter 5, the role of the navigator is to:

- Remove barriers

- Coach the patient and referring professional

- Organize key clinical and patient information

- Ensure that all appropriate tests are available to the specialist

- Act as a clearinghouse of key information

- Facilitate communication

The primary and support roles for navigation can be filled by clinicians, typically nurses, or by nonclinicians. The selection of such will dictate the responsibilities of the role. Staffing with RNs can provide additional capabilities, such as pretreatment patient education, review of posttreatment questions, and measuring response to treatment.

Software systems have been developed to assist in the navigation process to ensure specialist continuity, patient confidentiality, and coordination of care. However, although physicians understand that the current system is not working well for patients and for themselves, getting them to agree to have patients referred to an ITR system can be challenging. On the surface, they may feel as though they are losing control of the patient. In a well-coordinated ITR system, losing control of the patients is not an issue for physicians.

There are additional concerns about losing identity, truth in advertising, and the equitable distribution of patients based on training and experience. For example, a fellowship-trained spine surgeon who devotes 100% of his time to spine care does not want to be treated like a surgeon who devotes 10% of his time to spine care. Physicians who are faculty staff or spine physicians who work in one practice are the most amenable to implementing ITR systems. For private practice staff members in different offices, challenges in developing and deploying a centralized ITR system often occur because their respective interests are not fully aligned. It is important to align these interests.

Referral distribution

The process of equitably distributing hospital-generated referrals requires care, as perceptions of inequity can be corrosive to a collaborative spine program. Figure 10.4 captures, at a very basic level, the flow of patient referrals from the triage process and the referral to either surgical or nonsurgical spine specialists on an agreed-upon basis among spine specialists. Hospitals and physicians may develop criteria for participation in an ITR program beyond the mere ability to treat the spine patient. This may include training, hospital affiliations, and collection and sharing of outcomes.

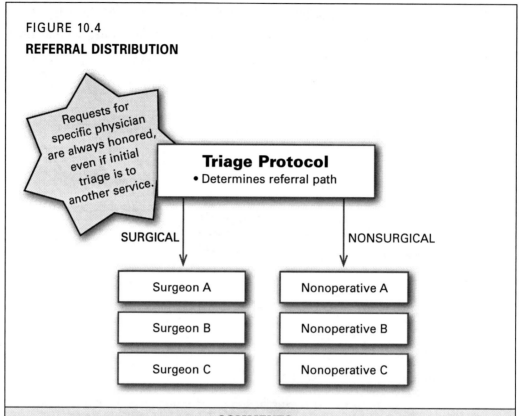

FIGURE 10.4

REFERRAL DISTRIBUTION

Requests for specific physician are always honored, even if initial triage is to another service.

Triage Protocol
• Determines referral path

SURGICAL

NONSURGICAL

Surgeon A	Nonoperative A
Surgeon B	Nonoperative B
Surgeon C	Nonoperative C

COMMENTS

• Hospitals and physicians establish prerequisites for referral (e.g., use of standard order sets, ED call, seniority, fellowship training, "live" schedulling, etc.)

• Establish and adhere to firm access standards: urgent = same day, expedited = 4 days, routine = 10 days, etc.

• Detailed protocols will need to be developed to address issues such as insurance coverage, availability of appointments within access standards, etc.

Patients who indicate a preference for a particular physician should be "tagged" with that participating physician at the point of intake. This patient will remain tied to this physician until he or she indicates a desire to discontinue the relationship or permanently refer to another participating surgeon. In this way, a patient who eventually may come to surgery will not be lost to that surgeon.

There are various methods for assigning surgeons. An example is provided in Figure 10.5.

FIGURE 10.5

SURGEON ASSIGNMENT METHODS

Method	Advantages	Disadvantages
Single rotation	• Guarantees an equal distribution among all physicians • Easy to administer	• Does not take clinical expertise or patient convenience into account
Appointment availability	• Ensures patients who require appointments will be seen sooner	• Difficult to determine on a daily basis
Group rotation	• Each physician group receives a similar number of referrals	• Disadvantages for surgeons from larger groups
Daily rotation or rotation tied to on-call responsibilities	• Surgeons can expect to review a block of new patients at one time	• Does not take clinical expertise or patient convenience into account • Not as equal as single rotation • More difficult to administer

In addition, the following factors should be considered when assigning surgeons:

- Geography/patient convenience

- Clinical subspecialty

- Surgeon's track record for reviewing patients in a timely fashion

- Insurance participation

Getting spine patients 'back on track'

A "back on track" diagnostic and treatment center—even a virtual one—is another must-have component specific to spine service lines.

After getting the right patient to the right provider in a timely manner, the next breakdown in the traditional system is often lack of coordination and follow-up. Providers are usually scattered in private practices throughout the community and are not linked together in any particular way. Spine specialists often do not know what has been done by the previous provider, nor do they communicate well with each other. Few, if any, actually record and aggregate the results of their interventions.

A "back on track" center or program has diagnostic and treatment capabilities and further coordinates care among providers. It is preferable to create a virtual center when spine care components exist at multiple locations but are tied together with common goals, a common identity, and a way to communicate information. The advantages of virtual spine centers are that office locations do not need to change.

Practices can maintain their own identities along with the "back on track" identity. The disadvantage of virtual spine centers is that they are typically not as patient friendly. Multiple locations make communication more difficult.

Actual or single-site spine centers work well when all or most components are brought together on an outpatient campus. A physical center creates a one-stop shop and can be easily branded. A center that provides quick access, coordinates care, and demonstrates quality results will draw patients, referring physicians, and insurance companies. Although having surgeons on-site is desirable, it's not essential. Many may prefer to maintain their locations with their orthopedic and neurosurgery group. Surgical patients can easily be referred to them at these locations.

There are challenges when trying to develop a physical center, including cost and alignment of clinical and business interests. Physicians who have been competitors are now being asked to partner. Meshing individually branded identities into one can be emotionally upsetting. Finally, aligning the priorities and business interests of multiple parties can be difficult.

There is no question that improving ITR, providing navigation, coordinating care, and measuring outcomes is the future of spine care. Hospitals and physician groups that are able to provide this level of service to patients will have a huge advantage over those that do not. It won't be easy to replace the individual provider model in favor of a coordinated patient-centric model. In very large multispecialty groups, this can be done independent of the hospital. But in most communities, the hospital must lead and fund the initiative. Hospitals with a strong private practice community and multiple providers should first consider development of a virtual outpatient spine center, with a long-term goal to develop an operationally and clinically integrated physical center. However, both models can be very successful if services are resourced, coordinated, and communicated to all constituents.

Spine center results

Although inpatient and outpatient spine care programs are complex and challenging to implement, most hospitals and affiliated practices that do so find the effort worthwhile. Consider the following data that client hospitals have reported.

Quantitative:

- 12%–20% increase in surgical volume

- 15%–28% decrease in LOS

- 20% increase in patients discharged to home vs. rehabilitation

- $1.5 million in incremental surgical and nonsurgical revenue in year one*

- Increases in hospital-based referrals to spine surgeons*

- Significant increases in hospital-based referrals to nonoperative spine care*

* Based on intake center development

Qualitative:

- Standardized care results in:

  - Predictability for medical and hospital staff members in processes and patient care

  - Greater staff confidence in respective roles due to specialization

- Greater patient readiness for surgery and rehabilitation

- Significantly expanded market awareness of services via word-of-mouth marketing among patients and PCPs

Comprehensive Sports Medicine

The Centers for Disease Control and Prevention (CDC) reports that each day more than 10,000 people receive treatment in the nation's EDs for injuries sustained in sport, recreation, and exercise (SRE). This represents one of every five visits to U.S. EDs. The CDC describes these injuries—which do not include other musculoskeletal injuries sustained in accidents, on the job, or in the home—as a "public health burden."[1]

Patients who go to the ED are seeking acute care that they perceive as not being available by other means. In the ED, they are evaluated, stabilized, and referred for definitive care as needed. Depending on the severity of injury, many patients are not referred, or they may lack the resources or resolve to pursue additional visits/treatments once a significant problem is ruled out. As a result, the ED is the only point at which the patient may receive such care, and this care, although adequate, is limited by the nature of the services available. There is a need to identify models that will provide more efficient and comprehensive care that will improve the treatment of the musculoskeletal-injured patient. The destination sports center can begin to address care for these patients.

The hospital is uniquely positioned to establish such a program because it is an institution that holds the public trust and has a reputation in the community as the leader for medical and injury care. The hospital either has the specialist resources for the program or can establish formal partnerships with various professionals for needed services in the community. These partnerships might include orthopedic surgeons, rehab providers, and training professionals, to name a few. The goal is to establish a core of sports medicine specialists to support a comprehensive program.

The clientele for sports medicine is not limited to athletes per se. It can include individuals of all ages who pursue sport, recreation, or exercise at any level, from elite competitors to weekend warriors to individuals increasing their activity to stave off other health problems. All of these "athletes" require the support of a comprehensive sports medicine program. Each seeks knowledge on training for performance and injury prevention, quick access to expert care for injuries, and rapid recovery programs that will minimize downtime.

Today, sports medicine programs exist in hospitals, training centers, and the offices of physicians, surgeons, chiropractors, physical therapists, and athletic trainers. Some providers may be fellowship-trained in sports medicine and/or have board certification. Others may simply declare themselves experts. Injury care is the primary focus, with prevention education following after the fact. Seldom will you find a comprehensive, coordinated sports medicine program that addresses injury prevention, education, and training; rapid access to care; injury assessment; and treatment that will support athletes of all ages and abilities in the community.

Such a program should strive to address the following patient concerns:

- How can I improve my participation and prevent injury?

- When should I be concerned about a pain or small injury?

- What exactly is injured and how can it be fixed?

- What caused this to happen, and was it preventable?

- Which treatments and interventions will get me back safely to my activity?

- How long will it take to get better? Will this be a permanent problem?

- Where can I turn for special education and services I need to for this injury?

- What should I do to prevent further injury?

An individual's sports medicine expectations vary greatly based on age, level of performance, and goals. The youth, adolescent, and young adult competitive athletes in organized sports seek to perform optimally and focus on the win. Others compete to enjoy the sport, recreation, or exercise and the associated health benefits. Each category requires guidance on training and injury prevention, but at different levels. All want fast intervention for injuries. They want to see sports medicine experts and receive care in a system that will address the problem quickly and efficiently.

The leadership, structure, and performance improvement team (PIT) for a sports medicine program are similar to those outlined in Chapter 5. Particular to this service line is the need to appoint a sports medicine director (SMD). The SMD position is designed to be both administrative and clinical. A physical therapist credentialed as a certified athletic trainer (ATC) or an orthopedic- or sports-certified specialist is ideal for the SMD position.

Initially, the SMD works to develop the scope and organization of the program along with the other PIT members. The SMD develops a standardized patient intake process and rapid recovery protocols, and identifies community sports medicine priority needs. It will be the SMD's duty, along with the hospital administration, to market the program to the network of PCPs, schools, community sports and recreation programs, and coaching and training organizations. After the program is developed, the physical therapist provides part-time clinical support in the hospital's outpatient PT clinic and on the sideline of identified sports events and serves part-time managing the service line.

The program's administrative lead also works with the SMD and the physician champion to define the scope of the program and build the infrastructure into the hospital. They coordinate on the many items that require oversight of the hospital leadership and are tasked to develop the business and marketing plans.

Popular services

A sports medicine service line provides basic training for community athletes and coaches. This can be done in three sessions per year, before the beginning of each season. Providing athletic trainers and physicians on the sidelines at high-risk events such as football games is important, but it is impossible to provide support for every event. This sport-specific and general training should be provided by sports physical therapists, ATCs, strength and conditioning coaches, fitness/exercise instructors, and so on.

Most hospitals do not have athletic trainers on staff. There may be physical therapists who are also ATCs or sports-certified specialists working for the hospital, but these providers are usually found in outpatient clinical facilities. The hospital must identify training specialists in the community to fulfill the program's training and injury prevention component.

These trainers may work independently or be employed by fitness or health centers. In these commercial centers, there is a varied scope of training expertise, equipment, and services. For example, trainers who specialize in adults may not understand the needs of young athletes. Therefore, multiple sources must be identified to meet the needs of identified high-volume athlete groups. The trainers must be carefully evaluated prior to establishing a partnership. The American College of Sports Medicine *(www.acsm.org)* offers guidelines on selecting and effectively using a health/fitness facility.

Sport-specific performance enhancement programs are growing in popularity. These programs objectively evaluate the athlete's strengths and weaknesses, design an optimal training program, and initiate a sports-specific exercise regimen, objectively tracking performance outcomes. Such programs may include gait labs for runners using video or mechanical technology.

The Medical Fitness Association *(www.medicalfitness.org)* is a nonprofit organization that assists in the development of medically integrated health and fitness centers. A hospital that develops such a center needs the public trust, along with the skill set and resources to address the sports medicine needs of all ages and levels. At these centers, profit can be realized based on self-pay memberships, similar to any other athletic club. These medically based fitness centers augment clinical services by extending the continuum of care through an array of fitness, rehabilitation (e.g., orthopedic, cardiac, and neurologic care), and tertiary prevention programs, such as occupational health and fall prevention. Eventually, the improved facilities for physical and occupational (potentially aquatic) therapy can generate more rehab referrals. This facility then becomes a magnet for other outpatient care, producing referrals to the hospital, its medical staff, and ancillary services.

Sports medicine specialists

The sports medicine program must identify and develop partnerships with medical professionals specializing in preventing, diagnosing, and treating SRE-related problems. The scope of practice includes musculoskeletal, sport-specific, gender-specific, acute, and overuse injuries, as well as medical/traumatic conditions affecting performance, such as diabetes, asthma, and concussion.

Depending on the medical discipline, this may include experience on the field, in the training room, the performance lab, the clinic, and, for the surgeons, in the OR.

 Orthopedics and Spine

The team may include sports medicine physicians, orthopedic surgeons, neurosurgeons, neurologists, primary care, musculoskeletal radiologists, orthopedic/sports physical therapists, athletic trainers, orthotists, chiropractors, exercise physiologists, psychologists, nutritionists, massage therapists, acupuncturists, and other related specialists. All of these individuals require sports training credentials that may include:

- Advanced training in sports medicine, such as that obtained by physicians, physical therapists, psychologists, and dietitians

- Board certification in the specialty and continuing medical education on sports-related topics

- Primary practice composed of at least 50% sports medicine

- Membership in organizations in which sports, exercise, fitness, and training are the primary interest

Rapid access to care

A cornerstone of a successful program is a system for expedited access to care that will allow the injured athlete priority appointments with appropriate specialists. Athletes do not want downtime, coaches require guidance on safely returning an injured team member to sport, and trainers and therapists need comprehensive understanding of the nature of the injury to start a recovery protocol. When children are injured, parents need reassurance that the injury will not lead to permanent disability. The system of access must accommodate all of these demands while taking into consideration the level of competition, nature of the sport, and type of athlete. Consider these guidelines:

- Sports with high impact probability and subsequent risk for injury, such as football, require sideline support. Identify community teams with need for game-time sideline support. Select sports medicine provider partners who will support the various events.

- Injured athletes need expedited access to care within 24–48 hours for non-emergent injuries. A sports injury hotline and/or a hospital Web appointment access system should be established. Intake information can be taken via phone or Web to allow for appropriate referral to participating providers. This intake information might include the location of problem, cause of injury, and onset time, as well as other demographics, such as name, age, and insurance information. Coaches and athletes working with specific team physicians will use a fast-track appointment system for competitive athletes. In communities where there is only one group, a hotline number may direct callers to the orthopedic surgeon's office. In communities where there are multiple providers, it could connect to the hospital.

- Rapid access also means a coordinated one-stop shop for the athlete. Multiple appointments for diagnosis and treatment—to the PCP, radiology, then an often-delayed specialist appointment—dissatisfies patients. The athlete wants to come for an evaluation, have imaging services and interpretation, bracing if necessary, and schedule rehab appointments all in the same visit.

A sports program must have all these services available promptly and at convenient times. The Shelbourne Knee Clinic at Methodist Hospital in Indianapolis is an example of a program in which the surgeon and therapist work side by side as a team to evaluate patients efficiently. The therapist initially screens the patients, performing the intake history and injury assessment, and begins to initiate basic treatment and education as appropriate. At the same visit, the surgeon reviews all intake information, evaluates the patient, orders additional tests as appropriate, makes the final diagnosis, and prescribes the treatment course. The therapist completes the final teaching and exercise recommendations.

If surgery is needed, it is scheduled the same day, along with the follow-up physician and rehab appointments. This coordinated team approach relies on a standardized patient flow process and trusted physician-therapist working relationship. The injured athlete leaves the clinic with a diagnosis, clear plan of care, an exercise plan and prescription, and education on physical limitations. This is all done in one visit. Follow-up appointments with the physician and therapist are set up as needed. The athletes can take the information to their coaches and trainers to plan for a safe return to sport.

Rapid recovery programs

Professional athletes must start treatment immediately following acute injury assessment. The surgeon and therapist must develop standardized rehab protocols for high-volume, high-risk procedures that guide and progress the athlete from the acute phase to the return to sport. Exercises, repetitions, and progression all should be outlined for the specific injury and procedure, along with acceptable cross-training methods. These protocols must be reviewed annually and updated in the PIT meeting of participating physicians and therapists.

Many athletes stop rehab treatment after the acute phase of therapy, often due to limited insurance coverage. Even with insurance, many patients use fewer PT appointments than necessary because of the expense of copays. In this case, the athlete is left on his or her own to progress to the return to full participation. Although this may be acceptable in some situations, it is not ideal. For those athletes who do not have trainer access, an alternative might be established, such as the creation of participation agreements with therapy providers to allow continued workout in the rehab facility for a fixed, reasonable fee. The rehab facility can offer specific times for athletes to advance their rehab independently in the clinic. They will have continued access to the equipment and the occasional counsel of a therapist to guide their progress to full recovery and address any problems that arise.

Outcomes measurement

As with all service lines, measuring your outcomes will set you apart from the competition. And in sports medicine, this data will help you obtain partnerships with resources such as physicians, surgeons, radiologists, therapists, dietitians, and psychologists in the community.

Functional outcomes should be collected, analyzed, reported, and discussed by the medical team. Did the patient return to sports? How long did it take? Only through an honest and objective look at the patient experience and performance outcomes can we be assured we are providing the best interventions and obtaining optimal results. Data analyses will either validate a program component or indicate performance problems that must be addressed. There may also be differences in outcomes among providers. The time and effort invested in gathering objective knowledge will pay the best return for the patients and their support team, providers, and the hospital.

Ideally, baseline metrics should be collected on all youth competitive athletes. Many sports medicine practices perform preseason physicals for athletes. Usually there is a standard form that is used, which gives medical clearance for participation. Seldom is there a basic performance assessment performed: how high the athlete jumps off the right and left legs; how fast the person runs 50 yards; or other simple tests specific to the sport. After sustaining an injury, these baseline performance metrics will give athletes goals to attain after injury and an understanding that just because the injury does not hurt anymore, it does not mean they are ready to return to full sport.

The payoff

Sports medicine is the gateway to musculoskeletal patients. Sports programs that are supported and branded by the hospital will be more comprehensive and likely more successful. As with spine care, both virtual and actual programs can thrive. Forward-looking hospitals should find a way to work with their physicians to include sports medicine into their orthopedic service lines.

Hand Centers

The hand is one of our primary instruments of discovery, commerce, communication, and personality. The loss of hand function or even the disfigurement of a hand can be disabling physically and emotionally. Hand injuries and disorders remain one of the most common reasons for diminished productivity or lost days at work.

For all of these reasons, it becomes obvious why developing a comprehensive clinical service in caring for the hand and upper extremity is important.

Unlike total joint, spine, and sports medicine services, true hand centers are not ubiquitous. All orthopedic and plastic surgeons have some training in hand surgery. Hand is a subspecialty that provides certification called a certificate of additional qualifications (CAQ), the first subspecialty of its kind to develop such a certification.

Many orthopedic and plastic surgery practices offer basic care for emergent and some elective hand and upper extremity problems, such as carpal tunnel syndrome, trigger finger, and other tendinopathies and tennis elbow. The care of these isolated injuries or disorders can be performed in most practice settings without additional dedicated support services. Most hospitals offer emergency services that include some hand care because of the high percentage of ED visits that are hand-related.

Practices that boast a fellowship-trained hand surgeon may offer a more comprehensive portfolio of diagnostic and surgical services for the hand, wrist, elbow, and shoulder, as well as on-site orthotics, prosthetics, and hand therapy. However, mostly due to the arduous emergency call demands of this subspecialty, a successful single-practitioner or even two-member hand surgery program is rare. Care delivery in hand surgery tends to be binary: Either the generalist does some basic hand work or a regional nuclear program provides access to three or four dedicated hand specialists to cover call and offer a full spectrum of surgical capabilities.

Hand surgery, which includes surgery of the hand and entire upper extremity, is performed for patients of all ages, both genders, and with all possible types of injury (e.g., traumatic, degenerative, metabolic, congenital, and neoplastic) affecting this anatomic region. Like the rest of orthopedics, the baby boom demographic will be driving many patient visits and surgeries.

Although some elective procedures, such as total elbow and shoulders, may be performed in a hospital setting and might require a hospital stay, most surgical procedures and diagnostic tests, such as MRI and nerve conduction tests, are done in outpatient settings. If the hospital can capture the revenue for these services, the benefit can be substantial. A considerable additional revenue stream may be generated by formalized hand rehabilitation therapy, which is an integral part of care for surgical and nonsurgical patients.

Because many orthopedic groups don't have an experienced hand surgeon on staff, they tend to refer patients in need of hand-related care to comprehensive hand centers. Despite the challenges of offering hand surgery, including a high number of workers' comp cases, creating a hand center will prevent you from losing patients permanently to centers with overlapping capabilities. Hospitals with a regional population base of 25,000–50,000 and a demographic rich in active 18- to 55-year-olds are likely to be in a good market to create hand centers.

Marketability

The public seems to harbor a fascination with the hand, with the press eager to report on powerful and interesting cases. Considerable free publicity will result from cases involving severe accidents or extreme success. For example, replantation of fingers or an entire hand almost always garners local or regional coverage. Seasonal injuries due to lawnmowers or snowblowers engage the community in a discourse about safety. In recent years, the busiest surgeons affiliated with professional sports teams have been the hand surgeons, creating a natural path for hand centers to brand themselves as destination centers for athletes, too.

All of these opportunities can create a halo effect for your entire facility. Because of the highly technical nature of the specialty, the public often associates hand surgeries with state-of-the-art facilities and capabilities.

Development and implementation

The approach to the development of a hand center is similar to that of the other subspecialty centers. Creating the right structure, leadership, and accountability is essential to effective management, optimal care delivery, and maximum profitability. Management needs to have the tools to organize and execute, and the surgeons need to feel enfranchised and efficient. As described in Chapter 5, the leadership team should include an identified surgeon champion, administrator, and program manager.

Further, your PIT should consist of representatives from every department that has contact with patients, including the following individuals:

- Engaged surgeons

- Anesthesiologists (with regional anesthesia experience)

- Physical/occupational therapists

- Social workers

- Financial counselors and workers' compensation experts

  Orthopedics and Spine

- Identified marketing/PR contacts

- Administration

Three models

There are three common models for creating hand centers:

- **Physician-owned center.** In some cases, a group of surgeons, and perhaps a neurologist, band together to form a hand center. Such centers are not affiliated with any one hospital and have multiple locations throughout an area. They often have their own outpatient surgery and hand therapy centers. This can be a highly effective model, but affiliation with a hospital is almost a requirement because of the high volume of emergency-related business that would fuel the practice. This low-overhead, lean alternative is attractive but requires constant vigilance and a combination of strong leadership and ultimate trust among constituents, which is sometimes difficult to generate or maintain.

- **Hospital-affiliated virtual center.** In this model, two or more private practice hand surgeons share space with an established hospital-based center. This is a complex model that often struggles with initial organization or sustainability because of the highly orchestrated fashion in which it must be administered and the difficulty in allocating resources equitably. The advantages to this approach are that it requires very little disruption to practice patterns and business relationships of the community of surgeons. However, there tends to be very little glue to hold such an enterprise together. This concept has success only when the surgeon's ability to render care or fiscally benefit by working alongside a competitor is considerably enhanced.

- **Hospital-based comprehensive hand center.** The true comprehensive hand center model places surgical specialists in an environment that includes all diagnostic and treatment modalities, plus laboratories and teaching facilities. Although these accoutrements can be dispersed among satellites, there should exist an identifiable nuclear location with dedicated resources and branding. This is known as a "hub and spoke" approach. Although the financial structure may vary among participants, patients will view the organization as a unified entity. The following elements are essential to such a center:

  - Orthopedic and/or plastic surgeons with fellowship training or CAQ

  - Occupational therapists and other rehabilitation specialists

  - Orthotics and prosthetics

  - Imaging (plain x-ray, fluoroscopy, MRI optional)

  - Electrodiagnostics

  - Electronic medical records

  - Work hardening services

Regardless of the model you choose, be sure to develop your hand center with the patient-centric model, described in Chapter 4, as your guide.

Hand center case study

The following case study was written in part by the center's director, Thomas
Graham, MD, whose work pioneered the specialty we know today as hand surgery.

THE CURTIS NATIONAL HAND CENTER & NATIONAL HAND SPECIALISTS PRACTICE AT UNION MEMORIAL HOSPITAL, BALTIMORE

In 1947, Dr. Raymond M. Curtis returned from service in World War II, where he was
among the initial group of surgeons convened to develop the specialty that we
know today as hand surgery. Enlisted by General Eisenhower and Surgeon General
Norman Kirk (an orthopedic surgeon), he returned to his native Baltimore and
announced that he was going to practice this nascent specialty.

Throughout the 1960s and 1970s, Curtis attracted other dedicated, like-minded surgeons to develop and perpetuate the legacy of Baltimore and Union Memorial
Hospital as the epicenter of hand surgery. The origins of today's contemporary hand
center concept are traced to Curtis and his colleagues building a service that included
diagnostic, therapeutic, and rehabilitation services all under one roof.

This 325-bed community hospital in Baltimore has not only become a world-renowned
hand center, but it has also trained 92 hand fellows from Walter Reed Army Medical
Center and 102 of its own Union Memorial Hospital fellows.

To put the contributions of this center in perspective, in 1994, the 103rd U.S. Congress named it the "National Center for the Care and Rehabilitation of the Hand and
Upper Extremity."

The center still values teaching as part of its mission but has grown to be a recognized destination for clinical excellence. It is located in its own facility and houses
one of the largest group of hand specialists found in one place. Approximately 70%

THE CURTIS NATIONAL HAND CENTER & NATIONAL HAND SPECIALISTS PRACTICE AT UNION MEMORIAL HOSPITAL, BALTIMORE (CONT.)

of the care is hand- and wrist-related, 20% rendered in the elbow, and 10% in the shoulder. About 35% of its cases are emergent in nature, and 65% are elective.

The center is of vast size and scope, boasting practitioners who concentrate their clinical and academic energies into the following specialty sectors:

- The athlete's hand

- The gifted hand (artists and entertainers)

- The National Arthritis Center

- Special hands (caring for children with congenital differences)

- The working hand (industrial injury prevention and treatment)

- The National Shoulder & Elbow Service

- The National Institute for Reconstructive Microsurgery

- The minimally invasive surgery initiative at the National Hand Center

The center's philosophy includes an emphasis on the patient experience and the need to receive input from patients and employees. Its goal is to be "locally dominant, regionally prominent, and nationally recognized." One unique characteristic is the desire to include other locally practicing surgeons in the activities of the center. As a result, hand surgeons from several other practices see patients, lecture, and take call under the mantle of the Curtis National Hand Center.

THE CURTIS NATIONAL HAND CENTER & NATIONAL HAND SPECIALISTS PRACTICE AT UNION MEMORIAL HOSPITAL, BALTIMORE (CONT.)

The right physicians

The hand center has 14 hand surgeons, including 12 orthopedic surgeons and two plastic surgeons, all of them board-certified and with CAQs in hand surgery. Each of them has articulated his or her philosophy of what it means to work at the center, educate the future leaders of the specialty, and contribute through scientific inquiry. Their insightful comments can be seen on the center's Web site, *www.nationalhandspecialists.com.*

Interestingly, only three surgeons are truly full-time at the Union Memorial Hospital base. The others devote 25%–75% of their time to practicing at the center, with the rest spent in private or satellite practice. All of them have taken call over the course of their career, and most still remain on the 24/7/365 call schedule that is one of the busiest of any service.

The right structure

The National Hand Center is led by hand surgeon and medical executive Dr. Thomas J. Graham. He is supported by a Union Memorial executive vice president, three assistants (executive, academic, and clinical), and a practice manager. He reports directly to the hospital CEO as well as executives of the Baltimore-Washington MedStar Health system, of which Union Memorial is a member institution. He is responsible for all aspects of the center, including clinical, academic, and financial functions.

The right thinking

The National Hand Center's triage system aims to get the patient to the "right surgeons, not just the next surgeon." The partners have a long history of collegial and collaborative thinking, which is demonstrated in the protocol to identify patients' complaints or problems and shuttle them to the subsection of the group that has articulated a desire to see those pathologies and/or has demonstrated special skills.

THE CURTIS NATIONAL HAND CENTER & NATIONAL HAND SPECIALISTS PRACTICE AT UNION MEMORIAL HOSPITAL, BALTIMORE (CONT.)

This is how the preceding list of specialty services makes a tangible difference in the patient experience and quality of care and is not just a marketing maneuver. The partners have self-selected their areas of concentration and constructed a matrix of care through which a patient may be guided to his or her optimal experience and result.

All of the hand surgeons are quick to point out the considerable positive effect that a close working relationship with hand therapists fosters. Not surprisingly, the therapists of the Curtis Hand Therapy Center literally wrote the book of treatments and protocols that have become the specialty's standard. This collaboration enhances the patient's experience and outcome immeasurably.

Dedicated staff and facility

The National Hand Center's 24,000-square-foot facility includes physician offices, clinics, the hand rehabilitation unit, a library, media facility, and even a museum. Other special areas, such as a fully equipped work laboratory in which almost every industrial job can be modeled, are fascinating amenities. Housed within Union Memorial Hospital are other Hand Center holdings, including teaching laboratories and a dedicated microsurgery skills training center.

As with a joint and spine inpatient program, having all the patients in one area offers the opportunity for patients to interact, receive emotional support, and motivate one another throughout the therapy process. This open concept was championed by Curtis and is looked on as one of his most significant contributions to the specialty.

The affiliation through a large healthcare system such as MedStar and its National Rehabilitation Hospital brand means that specialized hand therapy services can be accessed through any of the nearly 40 regional outpatient facilities.

THE CURTIS NATIONAL HAND CENTER & NATIONAL HAND SPECIALISTS PRACTICE AT UNION MEMORIAL HOSPITAL, BALTIMORE (CONT.)

Clinical services offered in the main facility include:

- Consultations with hand surgeons

- Management of acute or chronic pain

- Protective splinting for immobilization and controlled motion postoperatively or post-injury

- Exercise programs to restore motion, strength, and fine and gross motor coordination

- Home exercise programs

- Sensory reeducation programs after nerve injury

- Thermal and electrical modalities to minimize pain and swelling, facilitate restoration of joint motion and tendon gliding, and decrease hypersensitivity

- Whirlpools to assist with wound healing

- Patient education and instruction in adaptive techniques, joint protection, energy conservation, and work simplification

- Patient education in activity modification to prevent re-injury or worsening of condition

- Social work consultations

- Psychological help

THE CURTIS NATIONAL HAND CENTER & NATIONAL HAND SPECIALISTS PRACTICE AT UNION MEMORIAL HOSPITAL, BALTIMORE (CONT.)

Education and family involvement

Vice-chair of the Curtis Hand Center Dr. Hugh Baugher stated, "I believe the patient is best served if he [or she] understands as much as possible about his or her problem and enters into the decision-making." The center provides many educational opportunities for patients and families through multimedia applications and seeks consistent feedback on the success of the doctors' efforts to educate patients, even in regard to sophisticated concepts, such as hand reconstruction. Printed educational materials, videos, and books with pictures of surgical outcomes are shared with patients as they decide on treatment courses.

OR excellence

The 14 surgeons of the National Hand Center share nine ORs and dedicated staff members who are well versed in the instrumentation and protocols utilized by the individual surgeons. In addition, the hand service maintains three dedicated small ORs within the ED. These ER-ORs significantly improve the efficiency of patient care for this high-volume trauma service and serve to decompress the schedule in the main OR.

However, because of the large trauma volume seen at this regional referral center, the main operating facility also includes a dedicated trauma room.

Improving the patient experience

As partner Dr. Peter C. Innis said, "I am constantly striving to make the hand center more efficient and customer friendly. We strive for great service and processes to complement our great clinicians."

Dr. Graham has focused on hospitality-enhanced healthcare in almost all aspects of the center's operation and says it is one of major aspects of their success. As the

THE CURTIS NATIONAL HAND CENTER & NATIONAL HAND SPECIALISTS PRACTICE AT UNION MEMORIAL HOSPITAL, BALTIMORE (CONT.)

National Hand Center is the premier destination for the care of the professional athlete's hand and wrist, Graham has used the athlete's experience as a laboratory for identifying the germinal elements of an optimal patient experience. "The professional athlete is a great metaphor." Graham says. "They can go anywhere for their care, and they elect to come here, and they require 100th percentile outcome. What we have learned by treating that unique population has allowed us to enhance the experience and capability for all patients who come to the Curtis National Hand Center."

Teaching and learning culture

Teaching and learning have long been a core component of the center. The partners take seriously their charge to educate students, residents (Johns Hopkins, Georgetown, and Union Memorial), fellows, and colleagues. Conferences are ongoing and open to all physicians in the greater community, including a well-attended monthly journal club held in the evening in a relaxed atmosphere with dinner. One of the most impressive facilities is the surgical technique and technology laboratory, in which groups of up to 25 can dissect cadavers and exchange information.

Awards

In addition to its designation as the National Center for the Treatment and Rehabilitation of the Hand and Upper Extremity, the center earned official designation as the Hand and Upper Extremity Trauma Center for the State of Maryland by the Maryland Institute for Emergency Medical Service Systems in 2008. It is the only center in Maryland to receive the hand trauma designation and is one of the most unique specialty centers in the world.

Foot and Ankle Care

In nearly every community, you will see signs for foot/ankle centers, often within podiatry and orthopedic offices. For the most part, these centers offer diagnosis and treatment. Many offer pedorthotics and minor office procedures. Most of the surgical procedures are done in outpatient surgery centers.

The baby boom demographics that are driving huge numbers in joints and spine will be driving similar numbers in foot and ankle. Ankle replacements have improved and become a more common procedure. Patients are increasingly seeking out sub-specialists for care of their foot and ankle problems. However, the efforts to create a hospital-initiated foot/ankle center are worthwhile only if the hospital ensures that it can capture revenues from all services from diagnosis to surgery, meaning that it will have to compete strongly with office-based centers in the community.

Case study

The approach to the development of a foot/ankle center is similar to that of other centers. The following case study illustrates the principles found throughout this book put into action.

THE MERCY FOOT AND ANKLE CLINIC, BALTIMORE

The Mercy Foot and Ankle Clinic was established at Mercy Hospital in 2002 under the direction and vision of Dr. Mark Myerson. In 2002, Myerson left his large group practice to head up the clinic. His vision was to have a completely separate entity that would focus on foot and ankle care exclusively. He wanted academics and teaching to be a part of this vision.

The hospital hired Dr. Myerson and created a separate outpatient clinic in a building attached to the hospital. Initially, the space included nine exam rooms, two digital x-ray machines, two dedicated foot and ankle ORs, and a dedicated foot and ankle PT department. The department also provided diagnostics and medical products, including orthotics.

In the past seven years, the clinic has expanded from two surgeons to four and added a third OR. The clinic has three fellows and one weeklong international fellowship program. With 13,000 patient visits and 5,000 annual procedures, the clinic is busy and staffs 14 full-time equivalents, including one RN, one physician assistant (PA), two medical assistants, and three surgical coordinators. The PA is responsible for conducting history and physicals, some pain management, all hospital admissions, and some nonoperative care. Patient education is primarily provided by the surgeons, supplemented with booklets and videos.

The OR is heavily skewed toward major procedures, such as ankle replacements and triple arthrodesis, and averages 10 cases per day, running at about 65% utilization. Nearly all the patients are treated as outpatients, including some ankle replacements. According to Dr. Myerson and head nurse Dottie Devine, the following are the clinic's keys to success:

THE MERCY FOOT AND ANKLE CLINIC, BALTIMORE (CONT.)

- Alignment of physician and hospital visions over a 5- to 10-year span

- Complete focus on foot and ankle problems

- Mix of clinical, academic, and teaching

- Having more than one surgeon participate

- Nearly complete autonomy over the running of the entire center

- Extremely efficient OR, with seven-minute turnover times

- Nurses are salaried, not hourly, meaning they leave when work is done

- Quarterly production bonuses to staff members based on minutes in the OR (defined as cut to close) and number of cases

- Full support from Mercy hospital with little interference in the day-to-day management

Brian Cawley is the administrator of the clinic, among other responsibilities. Items such as billing and collections are handled by the hospital, as are HR issues, marketing, and PR. Myerson, Devine, and Cawley are a true team in managing every aspect of the clinic, OR, and patient experience.

Forty percent of the clinic's patients come from the local community and the employed primary care doctors that the medical center has deployed in strategic areas throughout the city. The other 60% come from outside the local community. As a result of Dr. Myerson and his colleagues' stature, orthopedic surgeons from nearly every state and country now refer patients to the Mercy Foot and Ankle Clinic.

288 **Orthopedics and Spine**

THE MERCY FOOT AND ANKLE CLINIC, BALTIMORE (CONT.)

Word of mouth is considered the key to the clinic's success. The team is very focused on providing every patient an excellent experience and making it as personal as possible. For example, the nurse who calls the patient the day before surgery will be the same nurse who prepares the patient for surgery and provides postoperative care. The same nurse then calls the day after to follow up with a specific set of questions that are aggregated and shared with the clinic staff. This creates a relationship with the patient and enhances trust. As a result, patient satisfaction scores are in the 90th percentile.

The clinic is also committed to collecting outcomes data. All patients, including those not part of research studies, fill out an industry-validated questionnaire before and after surgery. The scores are aggregated and used to identify progress and success. They have not yet been used for marketing purposes. Current marketing efforts include visiting PCPs appearing on television talk shows and publishing a clinic newsletter.

There are four employed podiatrists on staff at Mercy, three of them primarily non-operative. Efforts to include podiatry in the clinic have not yet succeeded, but an informal relationship exists between the foot/ankle clinic and podiatry. Some specific patients are referred to podiatry and vice versa.

Vision realized
Mercy Hospital used the star physician concept to develop its center. More importantly, this physician had a vision beyond himself to create a center that will thrive even after he leaves. As a result, Mercy and its physicians have developed a world-class foot and ankle center.

THE MERCY FOOT AND ANKLE CLINIC, BALTIMORE (CONT.)

Every aspect of the care, from the clinic to the OR to PT and orthotics, is focused on foot and ankle. The foot and ankle clinic is really a hospital within a hospital. Its mixture of clinical, academic, and teaching has made it the place to go for patients from around the globe. And yet staff members still provide simple foot care to everyone in the community and highly value the entire patient experience.

Not every hospital has the demographics to create such a comprehensive center, but the principles described here are still applicable. Smaller centers can be developed in conjunction with orthopedics and podiatry that can be focused, efficient, effective, and profitable. Leadership, a vision, and aligned goals are essential to success.

Summary

Every hospital, large and small, will need to develop subspecialty destination centers of superior performance if their patients are to enjoy the clinical benefits and hospitals are to realize the financial benefits of the coming flood of musculoskeletal patients from the baby boom generation. Great inpatient programs in joint, spine, and fracture care remain at the core of most hospital musculoskeletal programs. However, considerable benefits can be realized by working with your physicians to create equally appealing and beneficial outpatient programs in spine, sports medicine, hand, and foot/ankle.

Hospitals cannot do this alone. They need to create common a vision that will mobilize the support of all the stakeholders. They need to commit the resources to assess their current situation, architect a plan, implement it quickly, and assure that these programs achieve continuous improvement. With this accomplished, hospitals will have begun the process of transforming themselves and healthcare for the better, and be well positioned for the future.

Endnote

1. The Centers for Disease Control and Prevention, "Preventing Injuries in Sports, Recreation, and Exercise," *www.cdc.gov/ncipc/pub-res/research_agenda/05_sports.htm* (accessed June 29, 2009).

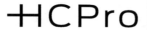